# Infant Intervention Programs:
# Truths and Untruths

The *Journal of Children in Contemporary Society* series:

# Infant Intervention Programs: Truths and Untruths

Edited by
Mary Frank, MS in Education

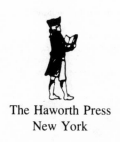

The Haworth Press
New York

*Infant Intervention Programs: Truths and Untruths* has also been published as *Journal of Children in Contemporary Society,* Volume 17, Number 1, Fall 1984.

The Haworth Press, Inc., 28 East 22 Street, New York, NY 10010

**Library of Congress Cataloging in Publication Data**

Main entry under title:

"Has also been published as Journal of children in contemporary society, volume 17, number 1, fall 1984"—Verso t.p.
Includes bibliographical references.
Contents: Early intervention and the early experience paradigm/Craig T. Ramey, Tanya M. Suarez—Prevention-oriented infant education programs/Donna M. Bryant, Craig T. Ramey—The efficacy of early intervention programs with environmentally at-risk infants/Glendon Casto, Karl White—[etc.]
1. Infants—Mental health services—Addresses, essays, lectures. 2. Infant psychiatry—Addresses, essays, lectures. 3. Child psychopathology—Addresses, essays, lectures. I. Frank, Mary (Mary Isabelle)
RJ502.5.I49 1984  618.92'89  84-22427
ISBN 0-86656-329-6

# Infant Intervention Programs: Truths and Untruths

Journal of Children in Contemporary Society
Volume 17, Number 1

## CONTENTS

### PART III: ISSUES RELATING TO STIMULATION
### AND CONTENT

## PART IV: COMMENTARY

# SELECTED READINGS

# Preface

The proliferation of infant research studies, infant intervention programs and newsstand literature indicates it is timely to examine critically the efficacy of infant intervention programs. In this issue an attempt was made to do just that.

To examine these programs, the issue was divided into three parts: The first part places our current thinking, research, public policy decisions about infant stimulation within an historical perspective. The paper also suggests the need for reconsidering our theoretical notions that underlie infant stimulation and suggests new directions to take with respect to the types of stimulation programs which are needed (Ramey and Suarez).

With this as a basis, the second part includes several articles that discuss the specific research that has been conducted to evaluate the effectiveness of the current intervention programs. Specifically, these articles focus on programs for the environmentally at-risk infant (Casto and White, McDonough), the developmentally delayed infant (Bryant and Ramey), and the handicapped or more seriously medically at-risk infant (Bricker). The final set of papers discuss the efficacy of stimulation programs by considering the more general issues upon which most programs are based. These include the problems associated with the various types of special programs (Honig), the biological development of the infant in relation to infant intervention, and, finally, general issues of normal child development as they apply to concepts of infant intervention (Brownell and Strauss). The last paper in this section is a commentary that attempts to explicate common issues that are discussed is a commentary that attempts to explicate common issues that are discussed throughout all the papers.

In summary, this is a "how-to-think" issue that is designed to elucidate the critical issues concerning infant intervention. It is hoped that these papers will stimulate some thoughts about the basic issues underlying infant intervention programs. While the issues presented here offer little practical advice for teachers and administrators involved in developing infant programs, it is hoped they will help to guide the philosophical base upon which quality programs are developed.

Mark Strauss, Ph.D., from the University of Pittsburgh contributed much time to the conceptualization of this issue along with contributing significant articles. The contributors, themselves all nationally recognized in this field, have also dedicated their valuable time to the development of substantive and thought-provoking articles. In addition, another behind the scene person is Linda Cohen from The Haworth Press whose skills and talents are ultimately responsible for the publication of this issue. We are deeply appreciative and grateful for the corporate efforts behind this ambitious endeavor.

*Mary I. Frank*

# Infant Intervention Programs: Truths and Untruths

# Part I

# PERSPECTIVES
# ON INFANT STIMULATION

# Early Intervention
# and the Early Experience Paradigm:
# Toward a Better Framework
# for Social Policy

Craig T. Ramey, PhD
Tanya M. Suarez, PhD

**ABSTRACT.** A model of intellectual development assuming direct and causal linkages between early experiences and subsequent intellectual functioning is seen as having constituted a basic but inadequate paradigm for developmental psychology. The predicted success of compensatory education was such a central tenet of the early experience paradigm that a failure to demonstrate permanent increases in intelligence with early intervention has constituted a basic challenge to the validity of the paradigm. It is argued that future evaluations of the efficacy of early educational intervention must recognize and go beyond the conceptual constraints imposed by the early experience paradigm with its emphasis on critical periods. A reconceptualization of the effects of early experience, emphasizing the cumulative and dialectical nature of development is advocated.

## INTRODUCTION

The beginning of Project Head Start marked an unprecedented commitment to the development of disadvantaged children. The major premise of Head Start was that systematic exposure to the basics

Craig T. Ramey is Director of Research at the Frank Porter Graham Child Development Center and Professor of Psychology and Pediatrics of the University of North Carolina, Chapel Hill, N.C. Tanya M. Suarez is Research Assistant Professor and Associate Director of Technical Assistance Development of the Frank Porter Graham Child Development Center of the University of North Carolina at Chapel Hill, Highway 54 By-Pass 071A, Chapel Hill, N.C. 27514. Preparation of this paper was supported by grants from NICHD (HD09130-10 and HD17496-02), Special Education Programs (G008300011), and ACYF (90CW602-03).

*3*

of American Mainstream Culture could boost the scholastic performance of children from socially and economically disadvantaged
families. Preschool education was chosen as one of President Johnson's weapons in the War-on-Poverty because it was implied by the
*early experience paradigm* derived from the *critical period hypothesis.*

Arthur Jensen (1969) rocked the intellectual and governmental establishment by publishing a forceful monograph which argued that
Head Start and other compensatory education programs had failed
because intellectual gains made during compensatory education programs eventually "washed-out". One response to the "wash-out"
criticism was the creation of a set of educational programs that began in infancy and which were more intense than Head Start. These
programs have been reviewed by Ramey, Bryant, and Suarez (in
press) and Bryant and Ramey (this issue) and will not be mentioned
specifically in this article. Rather, we will be concerned with the *rationale* for early intervention and its conceptual history. We will
conclude that the early experience paradigm is inadequate as a basis
for future compensatory education policy and must be replaced by a
paradigm which acknowledges the *cumulative* and *dialectical* nature
of development. It will also be argued that future educational
policies require research that more adequately addresses the biological, psychological, educational, and social *mechanisms* by
which experiences affect development.

## THE NATURE OF PARADIGMS

Scientific research is never conducted by unbiased researchers in
neutral environments. In contrast to the idealized picture of the ob-
jectivity of the scientific community, empirical research normally
takes place within the boundaries established by shared *beliefs* about
nature. Thomas Kuhn (1962) introduced the term *paradigm* to
define the pervasive models of reality that tell scientists about the
entities that nature can and cannot contain. Typical scientific research, according to Kuhn, is addressed to the articulation of the
theories and empirical phenomena that the accepted paradigms provides. The accepted paradigm defines the phenomena that constitute
valid research problems, and directs the procedures by which these
problems are addressed.

The study of human development, like other areas of scientific inquiry, is of necessity facilitated *and* constrained by adherence to a particular paradigm. So, too, is public policy affected by scientific paradigms. The paradigms that form the boundaries for inquiry into human development are particularly noteworthy because of their *immediate application* to educational practice and policy as well as to the conduct of empirical research.

The impact of a scientific paradigm on social policy is clearly apparent in the area of intellectual development and early education. During the past two decades, a model of intellectual development which presented early experiences as *critical determinants* of later intellectual functioning served as a guiding paradigm. This *early experience paradigm* provided the major theoretical rationale for preschool education programs designed to eradicate retarded intellectual development in children at high risk due to poor early environments. At present the early experience paradigm still specifies the criteria against which early educational intervention programs are evaluated. These criteria are (1) *significant* and (2) *permanent* alterations in intellectual and/or scholastic performance. In this way, the early experience paradigm has continuing ramifications for the future of research, practice, and social policy concerning intellectual development. For this reason, it is important to understand the historical background of this paradigm, and to explore the constraints on our understanding imposed by that viewpoint.

## ESTABLISHMENT OF THE EARLY EXPERIENCE PARADIGM

The idea that an individual's early experiences are of particular consequence for later development is an old one. Yet the significance of early experience has been advanced only intermittently in the history of Western thought. Other concepts have more frequently provided the dominant models of human development. In the 19th century, *predeterminism* was advanced by Galton and other proponents of the *primacy of heredity* in development.

Predeterminism, unlike the earlier notion of preformationism, acknowledged maturational changes in form as well as size, but held that these changes were relatively encapsulated and consequently unaffected by early experiences (Gottlieb, 1971). In the first half of the 20th century, the predeterministic view induced two empirical traditions that denied the contribution of early experience to later development: (1) the study of instincts as unlearned patterns of behavior, and (2) the investigation of behavioral development as controlled by the child's rate of biological maturation (Hunt, 1979).

The early experience paradigm replaced the concept of predeterminism in development with that of *probabilistic epigenesis.* While predeterminism assumed that the maturational process is relatively unaffected by experience, probabilistic epigenesis emphasized the importance of sensory stimulation and movement for subsequent development (Gottlieb, 1971). The early experience paradigm further held that the presence or absence of stimulation at *critical periods* in development could permanently alter the individual's developmental pattern.

How did the doctrine of the primacy of early experience come to be so entrenched in American psychology? Kuhn (1962) contends that both scientific and "extra-scientific" factors are involved in the establishment of any paradigm. Such was the case with the early experience paradigm; both the scientific and the political zeitgeist contributed to the construction of this model of reality.

## The Scientific Bases of the Early Experience Paradigm

Evidence from three major streams of investigations flowed together in establishing the doctrine of the primacy of early experience. *First,* Freud's theory of psychosexual development (1905) focused attention on childhood experiences and contributed significantly to the popular acceptance of the concept that early experience is a determinant of adult behavior. *Second,* ethology also contributed to the establishment of the early experience paradigm through the phenomenon of imprinting (Lorenz, 1937) which was interpreted as representing a unique predisposition for learning, present for only a brief critical period. The *third* scientific stream flowed from the work of Hebb (1949). He provided a neuropsychological theory for the existence of critical periods in intellectual as well as social development. Investigations with animals revealed that variations in early experiences affected both the *organization* and the *biological bases* of subsequent behavior (e.g., Thompson & Heron, 1954; Kretch, Rosenzweig, & Bennett, 1960).

As the early experience paradigm flowered, its roots branched from the Freudian idea that early experience is important for later social and sexual behavior to the belief that it is also critical for later human intellectual and instrumental competencies. Further, the con ceptualization of the impact of early experience was broadened and deepened. Initially, early experience was seen to predispose an individual toward a certain personality structure and a consequent propensity to respond to situations in predictable ways. Later, the extension of the concept of *critical periods* to humans from lower mammals conceptualized early experience as imparting stable and irreversible neurological consequences that could set a ceiling for later problem-solving behavior (e.g., Harlow, 1958). Although the empirical support for this notion was both scant and limited to investigations with laboratory animals, this interpretation of the effects of early experience formed the basis for much of the work done in the area of intellectual development in the past two decades.

The educational implications of this empirical background were assimilated in the works of J. McVicker Hunt and Benjamin Bloom. Hunt's (1961) "concept of the match" put forth in *Intelligence and Experience* was an application of Piaget's dialectical model of development and assigned a greater role in intellectual development to the characteristics of the environment than to the hereditary make-up of the individual. Developmental outcomes were seen as the cumulative result of the child's successive interactions with increasingly complex stimuli. Hence, adequate intellectual development depended upon the child's receiving appropriate stimulation at the appropriate point in development. Although Hunt's general thesis did not postulate critical periods in development, it implied that early experiences were particularly important.

In *Stability and Change in Human Characteristics,* Bloom (1964) made two major points that provided a major impetus for preschool intervention. First, he posited that intellectual growth occurred most rapidly in the first 4 or 5 years of life, and tapered off by the time the child had entered grade school. Second, Bloom argued that the first 5 years of life were a critical period for intellectual development. Intellectual development was, in his opinion, characterized by plasticity only during the early years of life. Consequently, the first few years provided the only opportunity for facilitating intellectual development by enriching the child's environment.

## Extra-Scientific Bases of the Early Experience Paradigm

The political zeitgeist of the 1960's was also an important influence on the public acceptance of the early experience paradigm. Public attention was directed in the early 1960's to widespread poverty and social injustice in the United States. In an effort to eradicate poverty while preserving the basic structure of the American economic system, economic deprivation was construed as cultural deprivation. The early experience paradigm was embraced by policymakers as a guide to social action. Early education was adapted as a paradigm-specified tool. This environmentalist viewpoint, with its emphasis on intellectual attainment in the compensatory education movement, harmonized well with the American spirit of action solution to a perplexing and pervasive problem.

Pragmatic concerns facilitated the immediate implementation of Project Head Start, the center of the compensatory movement and the embodiment of the early experience paradigm (Zigler & Anderson, 1979). As a service for children with a commonsense appeal, it enabled administrators to achieve program administration by the poor through parent involvement in program development without resistance from local governments, thereby facilitating the success of the controversial Community Action Programs.

## A PARADOX WITHIN THE EARLY EXPERIENCE PARADIGM

A strong emphasis on the importance of early experience in determining intellectual development involves the corollary that positive changes in the child's environment should result in increases in measured intelligence. This corollary formed the central rationale for the compensatory education movement. The early experience paradigm purported to identify the causes of psychosocial retardation and to specify the means by which it could be eradicated. According to the early experience paradigm, intellectual deficiencies arose from the inadequacy of the poor child's environment. These deficiencies and the resulting cycle of poverty could be eradicated by providing the poor child with compensatory education during the preschool years, the paradigm-specified critical period for intellectual development.

Operating within the early experience paradigm, a body of literature documenting widely-held beliefs and substantiating generally accepted theories was compiled through the 1960's. Yet, in spite of the selective attention and self-perpetuation of characteristics of a scientific paradigm, an anomaly appeared and persisted: Compensatory education did not keep its promises. A nationwide evaluation of

Project Head Start concluded that *no permanent benefits* from the program could be found. The positive effects of Head Start attendance, moreover, were fairly small in magnitude as well as apparently short-lived (Cicirelli, 1969). This pattern of results was also obtained in the initial evaluations of other early intervention programs (Bronfenbrenner, 1974).

The resulting attack on compensatory education inevitably became a battle concerning the early experience paradigm. Jensen (1969) argued that compensatory education had been tried but failed. He attributed depressed intellectual development in socially disadvantaged children to *genetic limitations* rather than to *environmental deprivation, a predeterministic point of view.* If the early environment could no longer be considered the prime determinant of intellectual development, then it must be that the genetic make-up of an individual is the critical factor. Thus, we are witnessing an attempt to retreat to an earlier but inadequate paradigm. What is needed, however, is to move forward to a more *comprehensive* and *adequate* worldview. We need a new paradigm to provide a more realistic set of expectations about human development in general and early education in particular.

## BEYOND THE EARLY EXPERIENCE PARADIGM

The early experience paradigm will, in all likelihood, be replaced by an alternative model of reality that will focus our research and policy attention and magnify our biases as effectively as the early experience paradigm. Science inevitably operates within paradigms. Any model of development is worthwhile only to the extent that it advances human knowledge and understanding. The early experience paradigm has left important legacies for understanding how science must look at human development. The shortcomings of the model have suggested some alternative routes to follow in better understanding human development.

## EARLY EXPERIENCE EXTENDED BEYOND PRESCHOOL YEARS

Seen outside a zeitgeist coercing an environmentalist interpretation, the empirical evidence suggests no simple model for the specification of the role of early experience in human development. Although some animal studies have documented direct and permanent effects of early experience on adult behavior, a more complex relationship between early stimulation and subsequent development characterizes ontogeny among humans. Human development proceeds at a much slower rate than does development among less highly evolved species. This may mean that *early* experience will have to be conceptualized as occurring over a longer period than just the preschool years. In addition, the effects of early experience may be increasingly reversible as behavior becomes more complexly organized and affected by multiple determinants (Hunt, 1979). For these reasons, the postulation of direct and necessary casual linkages between early experience and subsequent human development must be questioned. Clarke and Clarke (1976), for example, reviewed the evidence on the effects of early experience generally, and found that the hypotheses derived from the notion that the first years of life are critical for later development have not been supported.

## CUMULATIVE NATURE OF DEVELOPMENT

Only a rigid adherence to the early experience paradigm, however, necessitates the conclusion that early experience is unimportant for later performance. Recently, development has been conceptualized as a *continuous process,* a cumulative series of transactions between individuals and their environments (Ramey, Trohanis, & Hostler, 1982). This cumulative nature of development, rather than the existence of a critical period for the effects of early experience, still renders the early years of human life highly significant for later development (Ramey & Baker-Ward, 1983). The level of skills and competencies that individuals attain early in their lives affects their abilities to respond to later situations requiring adaptation and complex behavioral organization.

## DURATION OF EXPERIENCES

In addition, achieved, rather than potential, plasticity in development may be lessened by the tendency of society to associate particular experiences such as schooling with limited age spans, thus lowering the probability that certain developmental tasks will be accomplished after a specific time period. For example, an inferior early education might be mitigated by later superior education, but in reality it rarely is. Thus, the early experience paradigm need no longer constitute the pervasive model of intellectual development in order to justify early education.

## FUTURE DIRECTIONS

In order to advance our understanding of human development and to create sound and realistic educational policy for young children three types of research are now badly needed.

### Holistic Research

First, we need to recognize the contributions of environment, experience, and heredity on development, and to engage in multidisciplinary research to determine how these forces act in concert. Just as predeterminism gave way to the early experience paradigm, both of these worldviews must give way to a new paradigm that incorporates, but supercedes, both. Psychologists, educators, biologists, and physicians need to be brought together in teams to address developmental issues more adequately. The molding of these perspectives will enable us to stop the pendulum swing from nature to nurture and move to new insights into the processes that regulate human development.

### Mechanisms of Change

Second, we are in need of large-scale, social-action research which focuses equally on the mechanisms of change as well as on developmental outcomes. For too long we have evaluated early intervention programs solely on the basis of IQ gains. We need an equal focus on what aspects of educational programs cause developmental change and what, specifically, in the child and his family has been affected. Without a better understanding of change-mechanisms we are seriously handicapped in planning the next generation of early education programs.

### Timing and Duration

Third, on a policy level we need to encourage systematic research into the issues of developmental timing and duration of educational intervention. If we are to conduct sophisticated cost-effectiveness inquiries into alternative forms of early (and perhaps continuing) versus later (and perhaps briefer) educational interventions there is no adequate short-cut to systematic research. Thus, we argue for the necessity of multidisciplinary, process-oriented research which focuses on comparing the effectiveness of alternative educational programs and practices. Through such research we may even be successful in forging a new paradigm for understanding development and how to alter it positively if not permanently.

## IMPLICATIONS FOR CURRENT POLICIES

Until a better understanding regarding the nature and limits of early experience for practitioners is achieved, we recommend five guidelines concerning the operation of early intervention programs.

*First,* practitioners should assume that detrimental conditions will not change spontaneously and therefore at-risk children should be placed in systematic educational programs as soon as the risk status can be verified.

*Second,* high-risk children should remain in systematic educational programs until there is positive evidence that there has been a change in risk indicators for the better.

*Third,* particular emphasis should be placed on risk-indicators in the child's natural ecology rather than on the child's own cognitive or social performance.

*Fourth,* educators should try to involve parents meaningfully in the child's educational program to the limits of their ability to be involved.

*Fifth,* systematic variations in educational curricula and format should be tried with the aim of increasing both program effectiveness and client satisfaction.

## REFERENCES

Bloom, B. (1964). *Stability and change in human characteristics.* New York: Wiley.
Bronfenbrenner, U. (1975). Is early intervention effective? In M. Guttentag and E. L. Struening (Eds.), *Handbook of evaluation research* (Vol. 2, pp. 279-303). Beverly Hills, CA: Sage Publications.
Cicirelli, V. (June, 1969). *The impact of Head Start: An evaluation of the effects of Head Start on children's cognitive and affective development.* Athens, Ohio: Westinghouse Learning Corporation.
Clarke, A. M., & Clarke, A. D. B. (1976). *Early experience: Myth and evidence.* New York: Free Press.

Freud, S. (1905). *Drei abhandlungen zur sexual theorie.* Vienna: Deuicke. (Translated as *Three essays on the theory of sexuality.*)

Gottlieb, G. (1971). *Development of species identification in birds.* Chicago: University of Chicago Press.

Harlow, H. F. (1958). The nature of love. *American Psychologist, 13,* 673-685.

Hebb, D. O. (1949). *The organization of behavior.* New York: Wiley.

Hunt, J. McV. (1979). Psychological development: Early experience. *Annual Review of Psychology, 30,* 103-143.

Hunt, J. McV. (1961). *Intelligence and experience.* New York: Ronald Press.

Jensen, A. R. (1969). How much can we boost IQ and scholastic achievement? *Harvard Educational Review, 39,* 1-123.

Krech, D., Rosenwig, M. R., & Bennett, E. L. (1960). Effects of early environmental complexity and training on brain chemistry. *Journal of Comparative and Physiological Psychology, 53,* 509-519.

Kuhn, T. (1962). *The structure of scientific revolutions.* Chicago: University of Chicago Press.

Lorenz, K. (1937). Companion in the bird's world. *Auk, 54,* 245-273.

Ramey, C. T., & Baker-Ward, L. (1983). Early stimulation and mental retardation. In B. Wolman (Ed.), *International encyclopedia of neurology, psychiatry, psychoanalysis, and psychology.* New York: Van Nostrand Rheinhold.

Ramey, C. T. & Bryant, D. M. (in press). Prevention-oriented infant education programs. *Journal of Children in Contemporary Society.*

Ramey, C. T., Bryant, D. M., & Suarez, T. M. (in press). Preschool compensatory education and the modifiability of intelligence: A critical review. In D. Detterman (Ed.), *Current topics in human intelligence.* Norwood, N.J.: Ablex Publishing Corporation.

Ramey, C. T., Trohanis, P. L., & Hostler, S. L. (1982). An introduction. In C. T. Ramey & P. L. Trohanis (Eds.), *Finding and educating high-risk and handicapped infants.* Baltimore: University Park Press, 1-18.

Thompson, W. R., & Heron, W. (1954). The effects of early restriction on activity in dogs. *Journal of Comparative and Physiological Psychology, 47,* 77-82.

Zigler, E., & Anderson, K. (1979). An idea whose time has come. In E. Zigler and J. Valentine (Eds.), *Project Head Start.* New York: Free Press.

# Part II

# RESEARCH ON THE EFFICACY
# OF STIMULATION

# Prevention-Oriented
# Infant Education Programs

Donna M. Bryant, PhD
Craig T. Ramey, PhD

**ABSTRACT.** This paper reviews twelve experimentally-designed longitudinal studies of infant education. Without such early intervention, the disadvantaged infants who participated in these programs were predicted to become developmentally delayed. The interventions varied in their form, duration, and content. The major distinctions were between home or center-based programs and parent-oriented or child-oriented curricula. The magnitude of intellectual outcome scores seemed to relate to the intensity of the programs. Interventions that had more hours of contact with children and parents had more positive intellectual effects on the children, parents, and family life circumstances. Modest changes have been found in mother-child interaction patterns and quality of the home environment, although consistent measures have not been used across projects.

During the past 20 years numerous infant intervention studies have been conducted with infants from disadvantaged families, infants who were predicted to become developmentally delayed. The scientific and political reasons for this emphasis on infancy were described in the preceding paper by Ramey and Suarez. The purpose of this paper is to review some exemplary infant education programs, discussing both form and content as well as developmental

Donna M. Bryant is a Research Assistant Professor at the Frank Porter Graham Child Development Center, University of North Carolina at Chapel Hill, Highway 45 By-Pass 071A, Chapel Hill, N.C. 27514. Craig T. Ramey is Director of Research at the Frank Porter Graham Child Development Center, and Professor of Psychology and Pediatrics of the University of North Carolina, Chapel Hill, N.C. Preparation of this paper was partially supported by grants from NIH (1 R01 HD 17496-01), the Department of Education (G008300011), and the Robert Wood Johnson Foundation (7890).

*17*

and social outcomes. This review will be restricted to the published studies with preventive education for disadvantaged, at-risk infants who were randomly assigned to treatment and control groups and assessed longitudinally. We think that these studies provide the best scientific knowledge base from which to draw general conclusions.

First, a word about terminology. These programs are typically called infant *intervention* programs even though infants began the studies so early in life that they usually showed no signs of intellectual delay when they entered the program. Infants who were selected for these programs were typically those who were predicted to be at risk for developing later intellectual or social problems based on predictors such as parent education, income, or maternal IQ. By providing compensatory educational experiences these programs were really *preventive* in nature rather than remedial. Some infants, even at birth, have obvious special needs: low birthweight babies, for example (or Down's syndrome infants). Many different intervention programs have been studied with such infants, but few research studies using random assignment to treatment and control groups have been conducted with such clinical samples. For a review of this literature, the reader is referred to articles by Dunst and Rheingrover (1981) and Simeonsson, Cooper, and Scheiner (1982).

## OVERVIEW OF THE STUDIES

The twelve studies which met our criteria are listed in Table 1 along with one major reference for each study. All infants in these studies were from educationally and economically disadvantaged families and most samples were predominantly black. The three exceptions are the Houston Parent-Child Development Center (PCDC) study (Andrews et al., 1982) which was with Mexican-American families, the Ypsilanti-Carnegie Infant Education Program (Lambie, Bond, & Weikart, 1974) and the Family-oriented Home Visiting Program (Gray & Ruttle, 1980) which were more equally mixed black and white samples.

Other than the Houston PCDC study, no studies have been reported from West of the Mississippi River. Most of the studies were conducted in the late 1960's and early 1970's, a period when major social action programs were begun. This raises the questions of comparability of natural environments and the generalizability of the results to other communities or to current times. A few studies

Table 1

Characteristics of Infant Intervention Studies

| Name of Study | Primary Target(s) and Intervention Site(s) | Number of Subjects Entry | End | Child's Age at Entry & End of Program | Intensity | Activities |
|---|---|---|---|---|---|---|
| **Center-based, child and parent-focused** | | | | | | |
| Milwaukee Project (Garber & Heber, 1981) | Child and mother at Home and Center | Ea 20<br>C 20 | 17<br>18 | 3-6 months for child; 6 years for mother | Many hours of HVsb in 1st 4 months, then full-day daycare year-round | Children in educational program with a cognitive-language orientation in a structured environment using prescriptive teaching techniques. Vocational and social education program for mothers including job training and remedial education. |
| Project Care (Ramey, Bryant, Sparling and Wasik, 1983) | Child and mother in Center group (E1); mother in Home group (E2) | E1 16<br>E2 27<br>C 23 | 14<br>25<br>22 | 3 months - 4 years; project continues | Full-day daycare, year-round + biweekly HVs | Children in educational daycare program with focus on language and cognitive development and adaptive social behavior. All medical care provided. HVs to both E groups with focus on responsive parenting, learning activities, behavior management, and problem solving. |
| Carolina Abecedarian Project (Ramey, MacPhee & Yeates, 1982) | Child at Center | E 57<br>C 54 | 49<br>47 | 3 months - 6 years; project continues | Full-day daycare, year-round | Children in educational daycare program with focus on language and cognitive development and adaptive social behavior. All medical care provided. |
| Field's Center-Home Visit Comparison (Field, 1982) | Mother and child in Center group; mother only in Home group | E1 20<br>E2 20<br>C 20 | NRc<br>NR<br>NR | Birth - 12 months | Center= 20 hours/week; home =1/2 hour HV biweekly | Curriculum items modelled by HV; activities designed from the Denver and Bayley test items. Parent training in child development and in job skills via CETA employment. |

Table 1 (page 2)
Characteristics of the Intervention

| Name of Study | Primary Target(s) and Intervention Site(s) | Number of Subjects | | Child's Age at Entry & End of Program | Intensity | Activities |
|---|---|---|---|---|---|---|
| | | Entry | End | | | |
| **Center-based, parent-focused** | | | | | | |
| Birmingham Parent-Child Development Center (PCDC) (Andrews et al., 1982) | Mother and child at Center | E 162<br>C 89 | 71<br>65 | 3-5 months-3 years | to 11 months= 12 hours/week<br>12-17 months= 20 hours/week<br>18-36 months= 40 hours/week | To 11 months = Training in parenting and child development; mothers cared for own child with assistance from center staff. 12-17 months = 4 halfdays as understudies to teaching mothers; 1 halfday training in child development and family topics. 18-30 months = 4 mornings as teaching mothers, remaining time in training, taking care of own child, class preparation and social groups. |
| Houston PCDC (Andrews et al., 1982) | Mother, child and family at Home (Year 1) and Center (Year 2) | E 97<br>C 119 | 44<br>58 | 1 year - 3 years | Year 1= HVs for 30 weeks + 4 workshops; Year 2=4 half days/ week for 8 months + nightly meetings | Year 1 = HV topics in child development, parenting, home as learning environment, parent-child activities. Family workshops for problem solving and communication skills. Year 2 = Training in home management, child development and parenting; videotape and discussions of parent-child interactions. English classes offered weekly. |
| New Orleans PCDC (Andrews et al., 1982) | Mother and child at Center | E 67<br>C 59 | NR<br>NR | 2 months - 3 years | 3 hours 2 times per week | One weekly session to counsel on child development with 1-hour discussion group and 2-hour parent-child play experience. One weekly session focused on adult and family life. |

Table 1 (page 3)
Characteristics of the Intervention

| Name of Study | Primary Target(s) and Intervention Site(s) | Number of Subjects | | Child's Age at Entry & End of Program | Intensity | Activities |
|---|---|---|---|---|---|---|
| | | Entry | End | | | |
| **Home visit, parent-focused** | | | | | | |
| Mobile Unit for Child Health (Gutelius et al., 1977) | Mother and child at Home and in Mobile Health Unit | E 47<br>C 48 | 44<br>45 | From 7 months of pregnancy - 3 years | At least 20 medical and 24 infant stim. HVs over 3 years | Prenatal counseling; well-baby care; infant stimulation activities with emphasis on language; educational toy given to family often. 1st cohort received training on child development and family problems. |
| Florida Parent Education Project (Gordon & Guinagh, 1978) | Mother and child at Home | 3 yrs NR<br>2 yrs NR<br>1 yr NR<br>C NR<br>Total 309 | 24<br>35<br>83<br>50<br>192 | 3 months - 1, 2, or 3 years of age, depending on group | Weekly HVs for 3 years + playgroup for 2 hours twice a week in third year | HVs used infant stimulation activities with child and mother to help mother become more effective teacher of her child. Home Learning Center (HLC) in 3rd year, supervised by experienced parents, was a backyard playgroup for socialization skills. |
| Ypsilanti-Carnegie Infant Education Project (Lambie, Bond, & Weikart, 1974) | Mother and child at Home | E NR<br>C NR | 22<br>22 | 3, 7, or 11 months- 19, 23, or 27 months | Weekly 60-90 minute HV | Focus on mothers as teachers of their children. Piagetian-based formal set of infant activities to support objectives for mothers; emphasis on fine and gross motor skills. |
| Family-Oriented Home Visiting (Gray & Ruttle, 1980) | Mother at Home | E 27<br>C 20 | 20<br>17 | 17-24 months - 26-33 months | 30 weekly 60-90 minute HVs | Activities were based on DARCEE principles and materials for mothers of toddlers. Intervention tailored to each family, but emphasized teaching style, competence, language, and behavior management. Used inexpensive homemade materials. |

21

Table 1 (page 4)
Characteristics of the Intervention

| Name of Study | Primary Target(s) and Intervention Site(s) | Number of Subjects | | Child's Age at Entry & End of Program | Intensity | Activities |
|---|---|---|---|---|---|---|
| | | Entry | End | | | |
| Field's Home Visit Study (Field, Widmayer, Stringer, & Ignatoff, 1980) | Mother at Home | E 30<br>C 30 | 27<br>25 | Birth – 12 months | Biweekly 1/2-hour HVs | Curriculum items modelled by HV; activities designed from the Denver and Bayley test items. Goals to educate mothers on developmental milestones and to facilitate mother-child interaction. |

Note. The studies are arranged in categories in order of their apparent intensity of education as determined by hours of contact with children and/or parents. Within categories, studies are also ordered based on intensity as determined by hours of contact and/or provision of medical or support services.

aE = Experimental group, C = Control group

bHV = Home visit

cNR = Not Reported

22

have been conducted more recently. Both studies at the Mailman Center in Miami (Field, 1982; Field, Widmayer, Stringer, & Ignatoff, 1980) and both the Abecedarian and CARE programs at the Frank Porter Graham Center in Chapel Hill (Ramey, MacPhee, & Yeates, 1982; Ramey, Bryant, Sparling, & Wasik, 1983) were conducted in the late 1970's. Intervention is continuing for the Abecedarian and Project CARE children.

## Characteristics of the Intervention

Although it was difficult to summarize the complexity of the educational programs, we have attempted a capsule description of the characteristics of the intervention process for each of the 12 programs. Table 1 summarizes: (1) the primary targets of the intervention (usually either the child, the mother, or both), (2) the site of the educational intervention (usually the family's home or a child development center), (3) the numbers of subjects in the study, (4) the child's age at entry and at the end of program, (5) the intensity of the treatment or treatments within projects, and (6) a brief description of the educational activities as reported by the projects.

*Intensity.* The projects have been arranged in categories in order of their apparent intensity of education as determined by the numbers of hours per month that projects sought to have contact with parents and/or children. Within categories they are also arranged by intensity, with hours of contact and provision of other services (medical) taken into account. Typically, a center or school was the intervention site for the most intense studies. This is probably so because it is easier, and perhaps more cost-effective, for a child or parent to spend several hours in a daycare center than it is for a home visitor or teacher to spend several hours in one child's home. The most intense center-based programs, however, also included home visiting, thus attempting to alter the child's developmental course by changing the child directly and by changing parents' behavior and/or attitudes. Some of the most intense programs (e.g., the Milwaukee Project) also taught job skills to the mothers in an attempt to affect an even broader range of the child's environment.

Most home visit programs were less intense than center-based programs. They usually consisted of 60-90 minutes of intervention conducted once a week or less often. The least intense of these home visit programs lasted for a year or less. Weekly home visit interventions that lasted for 2 or 3 years would be considered moderately intense.

*Duration.* The duration of the most intense infant intervention studies lasted from birth until public school entry (the Milwaukee, Abecedarian, and CARE projects). Other studies intervened for only a year or two during infancy (e.g., the Parent Child Development Center (PCDC) projects, the Ypsilanti-Carnegie Project, and Family-oriented Home Visiting). A comparison of some of these studies based on age at intervention and length of treatment might pinpoint more definitively just how early and how long the "early experiences" have to occur in order to have an effect, either short-term or long-term, on intellectual development.

*Content.* All studies included, as part of their treatment, specific educational activities designed to teach the infant or child certain concepts or skills. These are summarized in Table 1. Depending on the mechanism targeted, these activities were either taught directly to the child (Abecedarian Project) or to the mother so that she could teach her child (Florida Parent Education Program). These activities were many and varied: gross motor, perceptual, language, adaptive social behavior, and Piagetian-based activities.

Many projects included curricula for parents in order to encourage greater parent involvement in the child's intellectual, emotional, and social development. The Milwaukee Project, Project CARE, the PCDCs, and the Mobile Unit project included parent training in areas such as problem solving, family life, and communication. Parent education occurred in large groups, small groups, or in one-to-one home visits. Field's Center-Home Visit Comparison and the Milwaukee Project included job training for the mother as part of the experimental treatment.

The activities conducted as part of the interventions were so diverse that it is difficult to make a general summary statement about treatments. Some treatments were described in a few pages or less, and some treatments used curricula that have been published and widely circulated. Most treatments were reported to be based on clearly defined theoretical models, yet the intervention was not specified in enough detail to determine that. It is clear that, even if we determine that some compensatory education programs have significant effects on IQ, little research to date has addressed the question of which components of the programs are most effective.

*Assessments.* Regardless of the educational philosophy, few studies assessed outcome based on the content of intervention. Standard developmental tests such as the Bayley and Stanford-Binet were the most common measures. The extent to which the scores from these tests are similar, especially for these samples of socially disadvantaged, primarily black samples, is at present not known. Data from Project CARE 2-year-olds indicate that Bayley MDI scores are consistently higher than Stanford-Binet IQ scores, but that the difference is greater for some groups than others. These results should be considered when interpreting outcomes.

## DEVELOPMENTAL RESULTS FROM INFANT EDUCATION STUDIES

The data base for the discussion to follow is composed of the mean Bayley MDI or Stanford-Binet IQ measures of experimental (E) and control (C) groups in each of the 12 intervention studies. These scores are presented in Table 2 where the studies are rank-ordered based on magnitude of E-C group differences in 3-year Stanford-Binet scores. Noting the size of the E-C differences is one way of indicating which interventions were most effective. Studies in which E children scored much higher on the Stanford-Binet than C children head the list in Table 2. Studies in which the groups differed very little at age 3 are near the bottom of the list. Standard deviations are not presented because they were not reported in some of the studies. In the two studies that compared daycare to home visit and control groups (Project CARE and Field's Center-Home Visit comparison), the scores of the most intense of the two treatments are compared to control group scores.

### Results at Age 1

A comparison of the nine studies that gave Bayley tests at 12 months indicates that the mean MDI scores of both experimental and control groups were unusually high for low socio-economic status (SES) populations presumed to be at elevated risk for slower development (E mean = 111; C mean = 104). The scores of the experimental groups were always greater than the scores of the control groups. In six of the nine studies the differences were statistically significant: (1) Abecedarian Project, (2) Project CARE, (3) Mobile Unit for Child Health, (4) Florida Parent Education Program, (5) Field's Center-Home Visit Comparison and (6) Field's Teen Home Visit study. In both of Field's studies the curriculum was based on the test items, so those differences might have been

Table 2

Intellectual Results from Early Intervention Studies Ranked by Magnitude of Experimental and Control Differences at 3 Years

| | Experimental Scores | | | Control Scores | | | E-C Differences | | |
|---|---|---|---|---|---|---|---|---|---|
| | 12 mo | 24 mo | 36 mo | 12 mo | 24 mo | 36 mo | 12 mo | 24 mo | 36 mo |
| Milwaukee Project | 117a | 125*b | 126* | 113 | 96 | 94 | 4 | 29 | 32 |
| Abecedarian | 111* | 96*b | 101* | 105 | 85 | 84 | 6 | 11 | 17 |
| Project CARE | 119* | 114* | 105* | 108 | 97 | 93 | 11 | 17 | 12 |
| Mobile Unit | 108* | 100* | 99* | 102 | 91 | 91 | 6 | 9 | 8 |
| Family-Oriented HV | | 89 | 93* | | 83 | 85 | | 6 | 8 |
| PCDC-Birmingham | 111 | 97* | 98* | 107 | 89 | 91 | 4 | 8 | 7 |
| PCDC-New Orleans | 111 | 101 | 105* | 107 | 100 | 99 | 4 | 1 | 6 |
| PCDC-Houston | 103 | 99* | 108 | 102 | 91 | 104 | 1 | 8 | 4 |
| Florida Parent Education | 111*c | 85 | 95 | 107 | 91 | 91 | 4 | -6 | 4 |
| Ypsilanti-Carnegie | 104 | 106 | 104 | 98 | 102 | 101 | 6 | 4 | 3 |
| Field's Center-HV Study | 119* | | | 106 | | | 13 | | |
| Field's Teen HV Study | 115* | | | 105 | | | 10 | | |
| Mean Bayley MDI or Stanford-Binet IQ | 111.2 (N=9) | 98.9 (N=8) | 103.4 (N=10) | 104.4 (N=9) | 93.0 (N=8) | 93.3 (N=10) | | | |

Note. All 36-month tests are Stanford-Binets.
All 12- and 24-month tests are Bayley MDIs except where indicated otherwise:
  a - Gesell at 10 months
  b - Stanford-Binet at 2 years
  c - Griffiths at 12 months
  * - Difference between E and C group significant at the .05 level or better

expected. Of the four remaining studies showing significant differences at 12 months, two were daycare studies, considered most intense, and two were home visit programs of moderate intensity. *Project CARE* (daycare plus home visits) showed an 11-point E-C difference at 12 months. The *Abecedarian Project* (daycare) showed a 6-point difference, as did the *Mobile Unit Project* (home visits plus medical care). *The Florida Program* (home visits) also showed a 4-point difference on the Griffiths test, which was statistically significant presumably because of the large number of subjects participating. With the exception of Project CARE, then, none of the infancy intervention projects showed a striking advantage for the treated groups by 12 months, perhaps because the scores of the control groups were still at or above average. Biological or maturational factors may play primary roles in the development of intelligence during infancy; the developmental process will occur if the infant is given at least minimal levels of sustenance and stimulation (McCall, 1981).

## Results at Age 2

Ten of the studies reported 2-year scores. Eight projects used Bayley tests and the Milwaukee and Abecedarian projects gave the Stanford-Binet. A comparison of the 2-year Bayley MDI scores indicates that E scores were greater than C scores for all studies (E mean = 99; C mean = 93) except for the Florida Parent Education Program. The Abecedarian and Milwaukee Projects used the Stanford-Binet which was also significantly greater for the E-group children than C-group children (E mean = 111; C mean = 91). In all, six of the ten studies reported that the E-C differences were statistically significant, indicating that the effects of the interventions on IQ were measurable by 2 years of age. Specifically, the early interventions did not improve Bayley scores for the experimental groups, but they prevented a large decline such as occurred in the untreated control groups.

The two projects which showed the largest E-C differences at 2 years were the two most intense center-based, parent-focused studies: (1) the Milwaukee Project (29 points) and (2) Project CARE (17 points). These projects also had the highest absolute E scores at 2 years (125 and 114, respectively). Both projects provided full-day, year-round daycare for E children as well as support services for the family, such as family education via center training and home visits. The Milwaukee Project also provided job training and placements for the E mothers. These most intense studies yielded the most dramatic results at 2 years. It should be noted, however, that the Milwaukee Project used the 1960 standardization norms of the Stanford-Binet, resulting in scores that are about 10 points higher than if the 1972 norms had been used; Project CARE used the later norms. The scores at age 2 would thus appear to be virtually identical for these two most intense studies.

Four other projects showed statistically significant intervention effects at 2 years, although the effects were less dramatic than those of the Milwaukee or CARE projects. (1) The Abecedarian Project (a most intense daycare program), (2) the Birmingham and (3) Houston PCDC studies (moderately intense center-based, parent-focused programs), and (4) the Mobile Unit for Child Health (a less intense home visit program that included medical care) all showed significant E-C differences of 8-11 points and absolute 2-year E scores ranging from 96 to 100. The Abecedarian Project was a full-day, year-round daycare intervention with fewer family support services than the Milwaukee or CARE projects. In type of treatment, though, it was most closely related to the most intense studies (the Milwaukee Project and Project CARE), yet in 2-year outcome it was more similar to the parent-focused studies, such as the PC DC's. Perhaps this was because the 1972 version of the Stanford-Binet was the test used at 2 years, whereas all other studies used the Bayley or the 1960 version of the Stanford-Binet. A 10-point increase in Abecedarian E and C scores would have resulted if the 1960 norms were used. These results would have been in the range (for both E and C groups) of the most intense intervention studies. Instead, Abecedarian results appear to fall in the moderate range.

The other three projects which showed moderate but statistically significant intervention effects at 2 years were parent-focused studies. Two of these studies were PCDC interventions at Birmingham and Houston (from the moderately intense group), which included extensive center training for parents. The third project, the Mobile Unit for Child Health (from the less intense group), was also a parent home visit program which included the provision of medical care, nutritional supplements and educational activities for the infants. Thus, two moderately intense and one less intense program showed significant intervention effects with E-group IQ scores averaging about 100.

The remaining infancy interventions—(1) the Ypsilanti-Carnegie

Infant Education Program, (2) New Orleans PCDC, and (3) Florida Parent Education Project—were all home visit programs and were relatively less intense than the studies previously mentioned. None resulted in statistically significant 2-year outcomes. The E-group Bayley scores of the Ypsilanti-Carnegie Infant Education Program and the New Orleans PCDC averaged around 100, but the C-group scores averaged around 100 as well. If these samples of children were at risk for developmental delay, it was not evidenced in the 2-year C scores, nor were the E scores significantly higher as a result of treatment. Gordon's Florida Parent Education Program also showed no treatment effect by age 2, and all E groups combined actually scored lower than the C group. The conclusion from these studies seems to be that weekly parent-focused home visits alone are not enough intervention to significantly alter the child's intellectual status by age 2.

Taken all together, the 2-year results from the infancy interventions support an intensity hypothesis. Home visits alone have not been shown to alter IQ by age 2. Home visits plus medical and educational intervention or parent-focused center training have moderate effects on IQ. Providing daycare plus other family services causes the most improvement in intellectual development. It is unclear which category of intensity encompasses the results from the provision of daycare alone.

### Results at Age 3

A comparison of the 3-year results from these infant intervention studies yields a rank-ordering very similar to that at age 2 and the studies seem to cluster into four groups based on 3-year outcomes. The Milwaukee Project, one of the three most intense treatments, showed the largest E-C difference (32 points), and forms a category of its own. The other two full-day daycare projects, Abecedarian and CARE, showed E-C differences of about one standard deviation, 17 and 12 points respectively, and form a second cluster. These three most intense studies, taken together, produced the strongest treatment effects.

The third cluster of studies based on 3-year Stanford-Binet scores includes, in order of intensity: (1) the Birmingham PCDC, (2) the New Orleans PCDC, (3) the Mobile Unit for Child Health, and (4) Family-oriented Home Visiting. These four programs had significant group differences, but the magnitude of the differences were 6,

7, or 8 IQ points, approximately one-half standard deviation. Two of these were moderately intense PCDC center-based, parent-focused interventions. The other two were less intense home visit, parent-focused studies. In our presumed hierarchy of intensity, the Mobile Unit for Child Health seemed more intense and lasted for twice as long as the Family-oriented Home Visiting Program, yet both had effects of 8 points. These latter two studies used different Stanford-Binet norms, but that should not have affected difference scores, although it may have affected absolute scores. The Family-oriented Home Visiting Program was the least intense of the seven studies which showed significant treatment effects. It was also the project with the lowest mean E group IQ, 93 points.

The fourth cluster of studies based on 3-year outcomes includes the three projects with no significant E-C group differences. These are: (1) the Houston PCDC, (2) the Florida Parent Education Program, and (3) the Ypsilanti-Carnegie Infant Education Program. In two of these three studies (Houston and Ypsilanti) both the E and C groups had mean Stanford-Binet scores greater than 100. In the Florida Parent Education Project, experimental subjects who participated in all 3 years of intervention performed significantly higher than controls; however, when all E groups were combined (including treatment groups of 1 and 2 years duration) the difference was not significant.

On the basis of the mean IQ of the experimental group children, the ten studies form two groups: (1) the Milwaukee Project (E mean = 126) and (2) all the other studies (E mean = 101, range 93-108). Given the range of intensities represented by the other nine studies, none of the E groups approach the high level of performance of the Milwaukee subjects. Even taking into account that the Milwaukee Project used 1960 Stanford-Binet norms, their performance still surpasses all the others, including the two full-day, year-round daycare projects—Abecedarian and CARE. The job training skills and experiences provided for the mothers by the Milwaukee Project in the first two years may have been a significant intervention above the beyond daycare and parenting skills. Given the potential strength of this treatment approach, it would have been very useful to have 2- and 3-year assessments in Field's Center-Home Visit Study because it also included job training.

All but one study that had significant treatment effects at age 2 continued to show significant E-C differences at age 3 (all but

Houston PCDC). In addition, the New Orleans PCDC and the Family-oriented Home Visiting Program showed significant effects for the first time at age 3. Patterns that were established earlier still seem to be present at age 3, although there were more changes in the E scores from 2 to 3 years of age than there were in the C scores. These changes are difficult to evaluate because most studies changed tests from the 2-year assessment to the 3-year assessment (from the Bayley to the Stanford-Binet).

## NON-COGNITIVE OUTCOME MEASURES

Because all of these early intervention studies administered Bayley or Stanford-Binet tests, they can be compared based on developmental outcome of the child. However, standardized tests of intelligence may not be the best way to estimate the abilities of disadvantaged children and such tests evaluate only one part of a child's functioning. Other measures have been used by various projects to broaden the scope of evaluation, but none are as standard as the IQ test. Assessment of mother-child interaction patterns and of the home environment have been the two areas receiving the most attention.

### Home Environment

Several projects used the Home Observation for Measurement of the Environment (HOME) scale (Caldwell & Bradley, 1966), a rating scale measuring interactions in the home and the quality of stimulation available to the child. The Florida Parent Education Program, Family-oriented Home Visiting, Field's Daycare-Home Visit Comparison study, and the Houston PCDC all reported increased HOME scores for their intervention groups, but only on some assessment occasions during the intervention period. Neither the Abecedarian nor CARE projects found HOME score differences between treatment or control groups. Other studies have used similar, although non-standardized measures. For example, the Mobile Unit Project reported significant increases in the frequency with which materials for writing or reading were available in the experimental homes. These home differences seem modest at best, and whether they last beyond the intervention period is doubtful.

## Mother-Child Interactions

Many of the infant education programs assessed mother-child interactions during play sessions or teaching tasks. Some significant differences were usually found in favor of the treatment group, but it should be noted that many statistical tests were typically conducted to analyze these results and the traditional .05 level of significance may have been reached by chance a certain number of times. Nevertheless, examples of these results may be instructive. For example, by 24 months, the E-group mothers in the Birmingham PCDC study held their children more, talked to them in a less restrictive manner, and used more praise. By 36 months the program mothers also provided more verbal information to their children. The E-group children were significantly more likely to play with, touch, or vocalize to their mothers than were the C-group children. The Houston and New Orleans PCDC studies found a similar scattering of results favoring the treatment group at 24 and 36 months.

The Ypsilanti-Carnegie Infant Education Program measured mother-child verbal interactions at several assessment occasions. E-group mothers in the home visit program engaged in more positive and facilitative language interaction with their infants than did C-group mothers. Although these differences were not maintained at follow-up, the verbal behavior of both mothers and infants was a significant predictor of children's later achievement test scores in school. The E-group mothers in the Family-oriented Home Visiting program used significantly more cue labels in their interactions with their children, a characteristic that was considered a good teaching strategy. E-group mothers in the Mobile Unit study conversed more with their children and handled their fussiness more appropriately than did C-group mothers; however, 48 other variables that were scored did not show groups differences. Lastly, the Abecedarian E-group mothers initiated mutual play more often and then engaged in mutual play significantly longer than did C-group mothers. Since there was no parent-focused curriculum in the Abecedarian study, these results were attributed to the fact that the E-group children were more active and verbal in modifying their mothers' behavior toward them than were C-group children (Farran & Ramey, 1980).

The mother-child interaction and home environment differences that have been reported have almost always been in favor of the treatment groups. These results serve as evidence of an intervention effect in these non-cognitive areas, yet the differences are usually modest and their enduring value is not known.

## Family Demographics

A more concrete and/or practical area in which intervention effects have been explored is that of family demographics. Field (1982) found that more of the home visit intervention teen mothers returned to work and fewer had repeat pregnancies. The percentages were even better among the daycare treatment group mothers. The mothers in the treatment group of the Mobile Unit Project also finished school more often. In the Milwaukee Project, E-group mothers' job stability and work performance were superior, and they earned an average of $40 per week more than C mothers. These "real life" results of intervention may, in the long run, improve the child's functioning by elevating the family's standard of living. The process through which this form of intervention might operate has not yet been clearly identified.

## CONCLUSIONS

The results summarized here are from assessments during or immediately following the intervention programs. Projects such as these are often criticized because their results seem to fade over time. Some of these projects continued to assess after intervention ended and some did not. The report of the Consortium for Longitudinal Studies (Lazar, Darlington, Murray, Royce, & Snipper, 1982) significantly increased our knowledge of the long-term effects of intervention. Specifically, children from the educational treatment groups were retained in grade less often in public school and were referred for special services less often. They performed somewhat better on achievement tests than controls, and they were more likely to give achievement-related responses to questions about themselves. Only a few of the Consortium studies, however, involved infants. A recent review by Ramey, Bryant, and Suarez (in press) indicates that intellectual benefits can be derived by children when compensatory education is begun at various points during the preschool years, at infancy, preschool, or kindergarten. Intensive educational programs may not be necessary in the first year of life, as long as good preschool programs exist to counter the declines that begin to occur around 18 months to 2 years.

This review of infant education studies seems to suggest that the more intense programs, those that had more hours of contact with children and included parents *and* children, had more positive intellectual effects on the children and on parent behaviors and family life circumstances. Practitioners should take this into account when designing new programs for children and their parents. If the realities of case loads or funding level prevent the practitioner from developing the ideal program, then creative solutions could be sought to increase the amount of contact with children or families. For example, the Frank Porter Graham program makes use of community volunteers who are trained and supervised by a psychologist. This increases the amount of one-to-one time available to the child. Other programs have relied to some extent on Big Buddies, YMCA volunteers, or "adoptive grandparents". It is difficult to find research studies comparing various types of volunteer programs, undoubtedly because it is difficult enough to conduct any one type of program.

An area for future research is that of program form and procedures. Program variations such as whether parents participate in group meetings versus home visits are probably more important than variations in curriculum content, such as Piagetian-oriented versus traditional didactic activities. Variations in the curricula that were delivered in these studies did not seem to account for outcome differences, although few studies have systematically varied curricula to determine differential effects. This would be a potentially useful area of research that would help practitioners interested in selecting appropriate curricula.

In summary, the studies reviewed support the general opinion that early educational experiences are important for children from disadvantaged families. At best, however, we can only expect modest gains, even from relatively intense studies. The outcomes of the projects reviewed do not point to any particular mechanism of change, to a specific intervention delivery system, or to a content of crucial importance. Our model of development must be broad enough to indicate that the infant's cognitive development can be affected directly or indirectly, through several sources (teacher, home visitor, parent, home environment), and across developmental periods.

## REFERENCES

Andrews, S. R., Blumenthal, J. B., Johnson, D. L., Kahn, A. J., Ferguson, C. J., Lasater, T. M., Malone, P. E., & Wallace, D. B. (1982). The skills of mothering: A study of

Parent Child Development Centers. *Monographs of the Society for Research in Child Development, 47* (6, Serial No. 198).

Caldwell, B., & Bradley, R. (1966). *Home Observation for Measurement of the Environment.* (The HOME manual is available from the Center for Child Development and Education, Univeristy of Arkansas at Little Rock, Arkansas 72204)

Dunst, C. J., & Rheingrover, R. M. (1981). Analysis of the efficacy of infant intervention programs for handicapped children. *Evaluation and Program Planning, 4,* 287-323.

Farran, D. C., & Ramey, C. T. (1980). Social class differences in dyadic involvement during infancy. *Child Development, 51,* 254-257.

Field, T. M. (1982). Infants born at risk: Early compensatory experiences. In L. Bond & J. Joffe (Eds.), *Facilitating infant and early childhood development.* Burlington, Vt.: University of Vermont Press.

Field, T., Widmayer, S., Stringer, S., & Ignatoff, E. (1980). Teenage, lower class black mothers and their preterm infants: An intervention and developmental follow-up. *Child Development, 51,* 426-436.

Garber, H., & Heber, R. (1981). The efficacy of early intervention with family rehabilitation. In M. Begab, H. C. Haywood, & H. L. Garber (Eds.), *Psychosocial influences in retarded performance.* Baltimore: University Park Press.

Gordon, I. J., & Guinagh, B. J. (March, 1978). *Middle school performance as a function of early stimulation.* (Final report to the Administration of Children, Youth and Families, Project No. NIH-HEW-OCD-90-C-908). Gainesville: University of Florida, Institute for Development of Human Resources; and Chapel Hill: University of North Carolina, School of Education.

Gray, S., & Ruttle, K. (1980). The Family-oriented Home Visiting Program: A longitudinal study. *Genetic Psychology Monographs, 102,* 299-316.

Gutelius, M. F., Kirsch, A. D., MacDonald, S., Brooks, M. R., & McErlean, T. (1977). Controlled study of child health supervision: Behavioral results. *Pediatrics, 60,* 294-304.

Lambie, D. Z., Bond, J. T., & Weikart, D. P. (1974). *Home teaching with mothers and infants: The Ypsilanti-Carnegie Infant Education Project—An experiment.* Ypsilanti, Michigan: High/Scope Educational Research Foundation.

Lazar, I., Darlington, R., Murray, H., Royce, J., & Snipper, A. (1982). Lasting effects of early education: A report from the Consortium for Longitudinal Studies. *Monographs of the Society for Research in Child Development, 47*(2-3, Serial No. 195).

McCall, R. B. (1981). Nature-nurture and the two realms of development: A proposed integration with respect to mental development. *Child Development, 52,* 1-12.

Ramey, C. T., Bryant, D. M., Sparling, J. J., & Wasik, B. H. (in press). Educational interventions to enhance intellectual development: Comprehensive daycare versus family education. In S. Harel & N. Anastasiow (Eds.), *The at-risk infant: Psychological, social, and medical aspects.* Baltimore: Paul H. Brooke.

Ramey, C. T., Bryant, D. M., Suarez, T. M. (in press). Preschool compensatory education and the modifiability of intelligence: A critical review. In D. Detterman (Ed.), *Current topics in human intelligence.* Norwood, N.J.: Ablex.

Ramey, C. T., MacPhee, D., & Yeates, K. O. (1982). Preventing developmental retardation: A general systems model. In L. A. Bond, & J. M. Joffe (Eds.), *Facilitating infant and early childhood development.* Hanover, N.H.: University Press of New England.

Simeonsson, R. J., Cooper, D. H., & Scheiner, A. P. (1982). A review and analysis of the effectiveness of early intervention programs. *Pediatrics, 69*(5), 635-641.

# The Efficacy of Early Intervention Programs With Environmentally At-Risk Infants

Glendon Casto, PhD
Karl White, PhD

**ABSTRACT.** The efficacy of early intervention programs for environmentally at-risk infants was examined using meta-analysis techniques. Questions relating to both short and long-term effectiveness and the influence of important variables such as age at which intervention begins, the relationship of parental involvement to intervention effectiveness, and the degree of structure in the intervention program were investigated. The analysis revealed that early intervention has an immediate positive effect of about one-half of a standard deviation. The analysis failed to find long-term benefits and failed to relate degree of parental involvement to intervention effectiveness. Some support was found for the notions that degree of structure and training of intervenor are positively related to effectiveness.

If one accepts the fact that from conception on, each individual is in constant interaction with the environment, and that at birth the infant is equipped with behaviors which enable him/her to interact with a favorable environment in a growth producing way, then the importance of environmental factors in the developmental process

Glendon Casto is Professor of Psychology and Director, Early Intervention Research Institute, Utah State University, Logan, Utah 84322. Karl White is Director of Planning and Evaluation, Exceptional Child Center, and Co-Director, Early Intervention Research Institute, Utah State University, Logan, Utah 84322.
Part of this paper was made possible by OSERS Grant #300-82-0367.

*37*

becomes apparent. In addition, even though infants may have great capacity for adaptation, the importance of the exchanges between the infant and the environment and the critical nature of environmental accommodation argue for some type of intervention when the environment is less than optimal. Environmentally at-risk infants are receiving increasing attention and programs attempting to ameliorate or prevent the impact of negative environments continue to proliferate. The environmentally at-risk infant is usually identified through the application of a risk index which includes such factors as parental education and income, maternal IQ, history of social/emotional problems, intactness of family, and need for public assistance.

Intervention programs have taken many forms, but the general intent of such programs has been to prevent the decline in intellectual development which usually occurs with these infants (Ramey & Bryant, 1983). The programs attempt to foster development in language, motor and social-emotional areas, and many times include nutritional components. The intensity of these programs have ranged from a few minutes of holding and cuddling a day for a few weeks to many hours per week of intensive intervention lasting for a year or more.

With the proliferation of early intervention programs, evidence has appeared attesting to their efficacy, and a series of review papers have promulgated conclusions which appear to represent the conventional wisdom of the field.

Statements such as the following are widely disseminated.

— The effects of early intervention are both immediate and long term.
— The earlier the age at which intervention begins, the more effective the program will be.
— Parental involvement contributes directly to intervention success.
— More structured intervention programs result in greater gains.
— More highly trained intervenors produce greater gains.

In an attempt to separate fact from fiction with regards to the efficacy of early intervention with disadvantaged infants, the Early intervention Research Institute at Utah State University has spent the past 18 months performing an integrative review of the early intervention research literature. Every research study which could be located was analyzed including studies using true experimental designs, quasi-experimental designs, and pre-post designs. This paper reports the results of this analysis and attempts to shed some light on the efficacy of early intervention with disadvantaged infants.

## LOCATION OF EARLY INTERVENTION EFFICACY RESEARCH

The following procedures were used to locate as many early intervention efficacy studies as possible. First, a computer-assisted search of ERIC, *Psychological Abstracts, CEC Abstracts, Dissertation Abstracts, Social Science Research, SSIE Current Research,* and *Index Medicus* data bases was conducted. Secondly, letters were written to over 75 infant researchers asking them to identify efficacy research which might not be reported in the professional literature. Third, previous reviews of the early intervention literature were examined to identify reports of efficacy research. Finally, efficacy reports referenced in studies already obtained were identified.

## PROCEDURES FOR CODING EACH EARLY INTERVENTION EFFICACY STUDY

A coding system was developed to analyze the outcomes and characteristics of each efficacy study identified. Based largely on an analysis of previous reviews of early intervention efficacy literature (Bush & White, 1983), variables in each of the following areas were coded for each study.

1. *A description of the subjects* included in the research (e.g., child's IQ prior to intervention, socio-economic status).

2. The type of *intervention* used home or center based, educational or medical.

The effect sizes included in the analysis came from studies conducted from 1937 to 1983, most since 1970. These studies were reported mostly in educational and psychological journals, but substantial numbers came from medical journals, books, ERIC documents, government reports, and dissertations. Many were unpublished articles. Not surprisingly, the most frequently measured outcome was some measure of IQ. Measures of temperament and motor skills, and such diverse outcomes as amount of mother-infant eye contact, weight gains, and various types of mother-infant attachment measures (Seashore, 1981) were also included.

3. The type and quality of *research design* employed, presence of various threats to validity and whether data collectors were blind. The quality of the research design was coded utilizing a one to five scale with one denoting a high quality study with a well executed true experimental design and five denoting a poor quality pre-post design with major flaws.

4. The type of *outcome* measured and the procedures used.

5. The *conclusions* reached by the study (the magnitude of the standardized mean difference effect size, the source of that information, conclusions of the author).

For each of the 97 items coded for each study, conventions or definitions were written. For example, the degree of structure for an educational intervention was coded using the following guidelines:

> *Very structured:* More than 50% of the intervention must be based on a detailed set of outcome objectives supported by a task analysis with scripted presentation of activities and procedures and criteria for progressing to new material.
>
> *Somewhat structured:* More than 50% of the intervention must be organized around preconceived activities based on explicit scope and sequence of learning. The relation of various parts of the curriculum must be specified and there should be the intention for interventionists to follow a preconceived, organized plan of instruction.
>
> *Not structured:* Any intervention which does not meet the criteria for 1 or 2 above.

The magnitude of the effect attributed to each intervention was estimated using a standardized mean difference effect size, defined as $(\overline{X}_E - \overline{X}_C) \div SD$ (Glass, McGaw, & Smith, 1981). This "effect size" measure is essentially the difference between experimental and control groups measured in standard score units, and has been widely used in recent years to describe the impact of educational programs (Cohen, 1977; Glass, 1976; Horst, Tallmadge, & Wood, 1975; Tallmadge, 1977). Using IQ as an example, an effect size of *one* would indicate that the experimental group scored 15 points higher than the control group. In cases where there was no control group and pre-post designs were used, the standardized mean difference effect size was defined as $\overline{X}_{posttest} - \overline{X}_{pretest}) \div SD_{pretest}$. In other words, when no control group was utilized, pretest scores were used as the best estimate of how subjects would have performed had they not received the treatment.

For some studies, there was insufficient information contained in the reports to code certain items. In those cases, the information was left blank. For example, it was possible to code type of design used for every study included, but the mother's educational level was reported or could be estimated in only about 30% of the studies.

It is also important to note that one study could yield multiple effect sizes. For example, a study which compared an experimental group to a control group on language and motor functioning immediately at the conclusion of the intervention program would yield two effect sizes, one for language and one for motor. The coding conventions dictated that only one effect size (ES) be measured for each 12-month period and for each domain (i.e., if two IQ tests were given during the same time period, results from only one of the IQ tests would be used).

Because multiple raters were involved in the study, interrater consistency checks were done for a sample of the studies coded (87% average agreement). Also, all Effect Size (ES) computations were independently checked, and a sample of keypunched data was checked against the original coding. More extensive explanation of the procedures utilized in the meta-analysis are available in Casto, White, and Taylor (1983).

## RESULTS AND DISCUSSION

### Characteristics of the Data Set

When the meta-analysis was completed there were 179 effect sizes computed from research studies dealing with environmentally at-risk infants (individuals who began intervention programs from 0 to 12 months of age). These effect sizes came from studies which compared intervention versus control groups and studies which compared one type of intervention versus another type.

The fact that early intervention efficacy research has focused primarily on measures of IQ is an important limitation which should be kept in mind when interpreting the results. Many important variables related to infant development as well as variables related to family functioning have been measured very infrequently. Thus, conclusions about the impact of early intervention in these areas are difficult, if not impossible, to draw.

## Overall Benefits

An overall summary of the data is shown in Table 1. As can be seen, the average effect size for intervention studies with disadvantaged infants was .43. This means if we consider IQ for example that the immediate effect of intervention was an average gain of 6-7 points for the experimental subjects over the control subjects. However, this is a somewhat gross estimate of early intervention impact. It is also important to break down the overall averages by various subjects and study characteristics. One basic breakdown is included in Table 1. As may be seen from the table, when the effect sizes are limited to only those which came from good quality studies, the average effect size increases. These overall results are the initial step in understanding the early intervention efficacy research.

## Long Term Benefits

The next important question is whether the benefits of early intervention are maintained over time or whether they "wash out". As shown in Table 2, the more time which has elapsed since the completion of the intervention program, the less benefit is observed. The average for 450 effect sizes measured immediately after the conclusion of intervention was .63. There was an immediate drop of ap-

Table 1

Average Effect Sizes for

Infant Studies

| AGE AT START | | | | | QUALITY OF STUDY: | | | | | |
|---|---|---|---|---|---|---|---|---|---|---|
| | | | | | GOOD | | FAIR | | POOR | |
| | $\overline{ES}$ | $S_e$ | $n_{ES}$ | $(n_{studies})$ | $\overline{ES}$ | $(n_{ES})$ | $\overline{ES}$ | $(n_{ES})$ | $\overline{ES}$ | $(n_{ES})$ |
| 0-6 MONTHS | .43 | .04 | 135 | (12) | .47 | (62) | .36 | (42) | .44 | (31) |
| 6-18 MONTHS | .42 | .07 | 71 | (14) | .55 | (22) | .30 | (25) | .44 | (24) |

Table 2

Average Effect Sizes for

Time of Measurement

| TIME OF MEASURE | $\overline{ES}$ | $S_e$ | $n_{ES}$ | ($n_{studies}$) | QUALITY OF STUDY: | | | | | |
|---|---|---|---|---|---|---|---|---|---|---|
| | | | | | GOOD | | FAIR | | POOR | |
| | | | | | $\overline{ES}$ | ($n_{ES}$) | $\overline{ES}$ | ($n_{ES}$) | $\overline{ES}$ | ($n_{ES}$) |
| IMMEDIATE | .63 | .03 | 415 | (69) | .51 | (121) | .61 | (128) | .72 | (166) |
| 1-12 MONTHS | .33 | .05 | 93 | (20) | .19 | (16) | .35 | (45) | .37 | (32) |
| 12-24 MONTHS | .29 | .04 | 75 | (23) | .33 | (23) | .28 | (27) | .25 | (25) |
| 24-36 MONTHS | .27 | .06 | 28 | (7) | .27 | (15) | .47 | (3) | .20 | (10) |
| 36-60 MONTHS | .02 | .07 | 52 | (8) | -.01 | (13) | -.02 | (30) | .17 | (9) |

proximately a third of a standard deviation for outcomes measured one month after intervention. The average for 135 effect sizes measured more than 36 months after the completion of treatment was essentially nil. The great majority of infant outcome measures were taken immediately after treatment.

The preponderance of the currently available evidence shows very little long-term benefits attributable to early intervention for disadvantaged infants. Of greatest concern is the limited amount of data upon which such conclusions must be made.

## *Programmatic Results*

As part of a larger analysis of early intervention with disadvantaged children which included all studies which began before 66 months of age, the effect of the following variables on intervention effectiveness was investigated (Casto et al., 1983).

1. Age at which intervention begins.
2. Involvement of parents in intervention programs.
3. Degree of structure in the intervention curriculum.
4. Training of the primary intervenor.

Although this data set includes studies which intervened with preschool children as well as infants, the larger number of studies, many of which are of excellent methodological quality, provide insights about variables which are important in intervention programs for environmentally at-risk infants.

*Age at which intervention begins.* A popular position in the early intervention literature is that the earlier a child is involved in a program, the more effective the program will be (Garland, Swanson, Stone, & Woodruff, 1981). In spite of its popularity, there is only meager support for this position. As shown in Table 3, the average effect size for intervention programs for disadvantaged children which began at different ages is very similar. When studies are limited to only high quality studies, there is a minor trend for programs beginning earlier to be more successful. For example, considering only the high quality studies, the average of 84 effect sizes in programs started before the children were 18 months of age was .50. Those 77 effect sizes which came from studies starting between 18 and 48 months was .37, and the average for the 25 effect sizes from interventions begun between 48 and 66 months of age was .26.

However, the results of an important study which made direct comparisons of starting children at two different ages (Gordon, 1969) showed only .08 of a standard deviation advantage for those children which began earlier.

From these data, it appears that although there may be a slight advantage for beginning intervention earlier, the advantage is not nearly so great as many people have assumed. Of major concern is the fact that so few empirical studies have addressed the issue of time at which intervention begins.

*Involvement of parents in intervention programs.* In early intervention programs for infants, parents typically take a major intervention role. That is, they are usually trained and provide a major part of the intervention in cognitive, motor, social-emotional, and language areas. One of the most frequent conclusions of previous

Table 3

Average Effect Sizes

For Age at Start

| AGE AT START | $\overline{ES}$ | $S_e$ | $n_{ES}$ | $(n_{studies})$ | QUALITY OF STUDY | | | | | |
|---|---|---|---|---|---|---|---|---|---|---|
| | | | | | GOOD | | FAIR | | POOR | |
| | | | | | $\overline{ES}$ | $(n_{ES})$ | $\overline{ES}$ | $(n_{ES})$ | $\overline{ES}$ | $(n_{ES})$ |
| 0-6 MONTHS | .43 | .04 | 135 | (12) | .47 | (62) | .36 | (42) | .44 | (31) |
| 6-18 MONTHS | .42 | .07 | 71 | (14) | .55 | (22) | .30 | (25) | .44 | (24) |
| 18-36 MONTHS | .69 | .07 | 93 | (14) | .35 | (7) | .63 | (26) | .75 | (60) |
| 36-48 MONTHS | .38 | .05 | 171 | (20) | .37 | (70) | .26 | (58) | .58 | (43) |
| 48-66 MONTHS | .33 | .04 | 264 | (22) | .26 | (25) | .49 | (88) | .25 | (151) |

reviewers of the early intervention efficacy literature was that programs which involve parents are more effective than programs which do not (Bronfenbrenner, 1974; Comptroller General, 1979; Goodson & Hess, 1975; Hewett, 1977; Weikart, Epstein, Schweinhart & Bond, 1978). Although this is an intuitively logical position, it is a position which is not supported from the available data. The average of 558 effect sizes from 56 studies in which parents were not used at all or were only used to a minor degree was .42. The average of 176 effect sizes from 20 studies in which parents were utilized as the major or only intervenor was .41. When effect sizes were limited to only high quality studies, there was still very little difference between programs which utilized parents extensively and those which did not (.40 versus .42).

Data from nine studies which made direct comparisons between different levels of parental involvement (Abbott & Sabatino, 1975; Bidder, Bryant, & Gray, 1975; Gordon, 1969; Karnes, Teska, & Hodgins, 1970; McCarthy, 1968; Miller & Dyer, 1975; Nedler & Sebra, 1971; Radin, 1971; Ramey & Bryant, 1983) were examined. When all 134 effect sizes from these studies were considered, there was a slight advantage for programs which involved parents more extensively (.08 standard deviations). However, these findings were heavily influenced by the Gordon study which found an average advantage of .18 for interventions which involved parents. The other eight studies found an average effect size of .06 favoring programs which did not involve parents.

Taken together, the data from these different sources of information suggest that programs which involve parents extensively may be effective, but they are no more effective than programs which do not involve parents. In other words, there is little support for the position that involvement of parents leads to more effective intervention programs.

*Training of primary intervenor.* When all data were considered, there was a substantial advantage for programs which used certified intervenors (ES = .47) versus those which used intervenors who are not certified. A certified intervenor would be an intervenor with a degree which would qualify one for certification in a professional field. For example, B.A. or B.S., R.O.T., R.P.T., R.N., and M.S.W. However, when the data set was limited to only high quality studies, these apparent differences largely disappeared (.41 versus .40). When the data were limited further to only those high quality studies which examined similar types of outcome measures (in this case, IQ), there was again a difference of approximately a third of a standard deviation. Those studies using certified intervenors found an average effect size of .63 for 51 different measures of IQ from high quality studies, while those high quality studies which utilized noncertified intervenors found an average effect size of .33 for 44 measures of IQ. Only three studies (Barbarack & Horton, 1970; Karnes, 1973; Schortinghuis & Frohman, 1974) were located which made direct comparisons between the utilization of certified versus noncertified intervenors (i.e., professionals vs. paraprofessionals). The ES's from these three studies showed an average advantage of .16 favoring professionals. Thus, the evidence with regard to the training of the primary intervenor is somewhat contradictory. Although there is some evidence to suggest an advantage for certified intervenors, it is weakened by the inconsistency of results when the data are analyzed in different ways.

*Degree of structure in the intervention curriculum.* For each study which utilized an educational intervention approach, a determination was made as to whether the intervention was very structured, somewhat structured, or had little or no structure. As shown in Table 4, the average effect size from 18 *very structured* interventions was .47. The average effect size from 37 studies utilizing *somewhat structured* interventions was .41. The average effect size from 15 studies using *little or no structure* was .30. Thus, there is a consistent decline in average effect size as interventions using less structure are implemented with disadvantaged infants and pre-schoolers. Similar but more dramatic results are found when effect sizes only come from high quality studies.

Two other findings of the meta-analysis are worth noting. The first findings concern the fact that many of the infant studies reviewed had high quality research designs with randomized assignment to groups. For example, studies done by Field (1980), Gordon (1969), and Ramey and Bryant (1983) are examples of high quality randomized designs. A second finding concerns a major problem

Table 4

Average Effect Size for

Degree of Structure

| DEGREE OF STRUCTURE | | | | | QUALITY OF STUDY: | | | | | |
|---|---|---|---|---|---|---|---|---|---|---|
| | | | | | GOOD | | FAIR | | POOR | |
| | $\overline{ES}$ | $S_e$ | $n_{ES}$ | $(n_{studies})$ | $\overline{ES}$ | $(n_{ES})$ | $\overline{ES}$ | $(n_{ES})$ | $\overline{ES}$ | $(n_{ES})$ |
| VERY STRUCTURED | .47 | .06 | 105 | (18) | .59 | (25) | .16 | (23) | .55 | (57) |
| SOMEWHAT STRUCTURED | .41 | .03 | 457 | (37) | .39 | (132) | .46 | (153) | .38 | (172) |
| LITTLE OR NO STRUCTURE | .30 | .05 | 77 | (15) | .12 | (12) | .44 | (34) | .21 | (31) |

for infant researchers, this being the collection of appropriate outcome data. As mentioned earlier, IQ measures were the most common type of outcome measure utilized. The utility of these measures is somewhat questionable because of the low correlation of infant IQ scores to later IQ scores. In selecting outcome measures, researchers might well be more explicit about outcome objectives, link outcome measures to these objectives, and be more concerned about relating infant outcome measures to the future developmental status of the infant population.

## CONCLUSIONS

### The Efficacy of Early Intervention

The results of the meta-analysis work thus far completed provide important information about the efficacy of early intervention for environmentally and at-risk infants. There is compelling evidence that early intervention for environmentally at-risk infants has an immediate, positive effect on about one-half of a standard deviation. Effects of that size are educationally significant. Equally important is that we know less about the efficacy of early intervention than has typically been assumed. Very little research is available to answer definitive questions about the effects of parental involvement, age at which intervention begins, setting, type of intervention, or long-term maintenance of effects. The data that are available frequently contradict the conventional wisdom about those variables (e.g., "the earlier the better").

### Future Directions

We should continue to provide early intervention programs for disadvantaged infants, but our goal should be to *design more efficacious programs. A first step* would be to use programs of demonstrated effectiveness as models for improving on current efforts. *A next step* would be to broaden the spectrum of outcome measures used to document efficacy.

We should also *intensify our research efforts* in early intervention, keeping in mind the lessons learned from previous research. Greater attention to *rigorous research designs* and *careful selection* of appropriate outcome measures can only enhance this effort.

# REFERENCES

Abbott, J., & Sabatino, D. (1975). Teacher-mom intervention with academic high-risk pre-school children. *Exceptional Children, 41,* 267-269.

Barbarack, C. R., & Horton, D. M. (1970). *Educational intervention in the home and para-professional career development: A second generation mother study with an emphasis on cost and benefits (final report).* Nashville, TN: Demonstration and Research Center for Early Education, George Peabody College for Teachers.

Bidder, R. T., Bryant, G., & Gray, O. P. (1975). Benefits of Down's syndrome children through training their mothers. *Archives of Disease in Childhood, 50,* 383-386.

Bronfenbrenner, U. (1974). *A report on longitudinal evaluations of preschool programs Vol. 2): Is early intervention effective?* Washington, D. C.: Office of Child Development. (ERIC Document Reproduction Service No. ED 093 501)

Bush, D. W., & White, K. R. (1983). *The efficacy of early intervention: What can be learned from previous reviews of the literature?* Paper presented at the annual meeting of the Rocky Mountain Psychological Association, Snowbird, Utah.

Casto, G., White, K., & Taylor, C. (1983). *Final report 1982-83 work scope.* Logan, Utah: Early Intervention Research Institute, Utah State University.

Cohen, J. (1977). *Statistical power analysis for the behavioral sciences.* New York: Academic Press.

Comptroller General (1979). *Early childhood and family development programs improve the quality of life for low income families.* Report to the Congress.

Field, T., Widmayer, S. M., Stringer, S., & Ignatoff, E. (1980). Teenage, lower class, black mothers and their preterm infants: An intervention and developmental follow-up. *Child Development, 53,* 426-436.

Garland, C., Swanson, J., Stone, N. W., & Woodruff, G. (Eds.). (1981). *Early intervention for children with special needs and their families: Findings and recommendations.* Seattle, Washington: Washington University. (ERIC Document Reproduction Service No. ED 207 278.)

Glass, G. V. (1976). Primary, secondary, and meta-analysis of research. *Educational Researcher, 5*(10), 3-8.

Goodson, B. D., & Hess, R. D. (1975). *Parents as teachers of young children: An evaluative review of some contemporary concepts and programs.* Stanford: Stanford University, Department of Psychology.

Gordon, I. J. (1969). Stimulation via parent education. *Children, 16*(2), 57-58.

Hewett, K. D. (1977). *Partners with parents: The Home Start experience with preschoolers and their families* (DHEW Publication No. DHEW OHDS 78-31106). Washington, D.C.: U.S. Department of Health, Education, and Welfare.

Horst, D. P., Tallmadge, G. K., & Wood, C. T. (1975). *A practical guide to measuring project impact on student achievement* (No. 1, Stock No. 017-080-01460-2). Washington, D.C.: U.S. Government Printing Office.

Karnes, M. B. (1973). Evaluation and implications of research with young handicapped low-income children. In J. C. Stanley (Ed.), *Compensatory education for children ages two to eight: Recent studies of educational intervention.* Baltimore: Johns Hopkins University Press.

Karnes, M. B., Teska, J. A., & Hodgins, A. S. (1970). The effects of four programs of classroom intervention on the intellectual and language development of 4-year-old disadvantaged children. *American Journal of Orthopsychiatry, 40,* 58-76.

McCarthy, J. L. G. (1968). *Changing parent attitudes and improving language and intellectual abilities of culturally disadvantaged four-year-old children through parent involvement.* Unpublished doctoral dissertation, Indiana University.

Miller, L. B., & Dyer, J. L. (1975). Four preschool programs: Their dimensions and effects. *Monographs of the Society for Research in Child Development, 40* (Serial No. 162, Nos. 5-6).

Nedler, S., & Sebra, P. (1971). Intervention strategies for Spanish-speaking preschool children. *Child Development, 42,* 259-267.

Radin, N. (1971). *Three degrees of parent involvement in a preschool program: Impact on mothers and children.* Paper presented at the annual meeting of the Midwestern Psychological Association, Detroit, Michigan. (Eric Document Reproduction Service No. ED 052 831).

Ramey, C. T., & Bryant D. M. (1983). *Enhancing the development of socially disadvantaged children with programs of varying intensities.* Paper presented at the American Psychological Association, Anaheim, California.

Ramey, C., Bryant, D., & Suarez, T. (in press). Preschool compensatory education and the modifiability of intelligence: A critical review. In D. Detterman (Ed.), *Current topics in human intelligence.* NJ: Ablex Publishers.

Schortinghuis, M. S., & Frohman, A. (1974). A comparison of paraprofessional and professional success with preschool children. *Journal of Learning Disabilities, 7*(4), 62-65.

Seashore, M. (1981). Mother-infant separation: Outcome assessment. In V. Smeriglio (Ed.), *Newborns and parents: Parent-infant contact with newborn sensory stimulation.* Hillsdale, NJ: Erlbaum.

Tallmadge, G. K. (1977). *Ideabook: The Joint Dissemination Review Panel.* Washington, D.C.: U.S. Office of Education.

Weikart, D. P., Epstein, A. S., Schweinhart, L., & Bond, J. T. (1978). *The Ypsilanti Preschool Curriculum Demonstration Project.* Ypsilanti, MI: High/Scope Educational Research Foundation, Monograph Series No. 4.

# The Effectiveness
# of Early Intervention With Handicapped
# and Medically At-Risk Infants

## Diane Bricker, PhD

**ABSTRACT.** A considerable body of literature on early intervention efforts with handicapped and medically at-risk infants exists.
Unfortunately, most of this literature addresses issues apart from
program impact or provides no objective evaluation outcomes. As-
sessing the impact of the efficacy studies that are available must be
done in the context of the constraints facing intervention researchers. Population variability, inability to execute sound designs,
differences in dependent measures and equivalent outcomes impede
the drawing of firm and generalizable conclusions. Nevertheless,
given these constraints many investigators and reviewers have concluded that early intervention efforts appear to produce positive outcomes on participating infants and their families.

As indicated in the title, the purpose of this article is to present information on the impact of early intervention programs on populations of handicapped and medically at-risk infants. An analysis of
the effectiveness of early intervention may assist the reader in determining whether the considerable investment of material and human
resources in these programs is defensible. Specifically, the intent of
this article is to discuss the reported impact of early intervention
programs on these two populations of infants and to draw conclusions warranted by the assembled data. As a necessary foundation for evaluating this efficacy research, selected background infor-

Diane Bricker is a Professor of Special Education and Director of the Early Intervention Program, Center on Human Development, University of Oregon, Eugene, Oregon
97403-1211.

mation will be presented. This information will include a discussion
of the problems associated with intervention research and a description of the elements common to most early intervention programs.

## LIMITATIONS OF INTERVENTION RESEARCH

Ferry (1981) reflects the frustration surrounding the evaluation of
early intervention efforts in her statement, ". . . the field is
hampered by enormous methodological problems." These problems include populations, measurements, designs, analyses, the relationship between dependent and independent variables and cost.

### Population Problems

Conducting intervention research with *handicapped* infants poses
several problems (Garwood, 1982). In comparison with normal and
at-risk populations, there are substantially (1) fewer handicapped
children, (2) more heterogeneous populations, and (3) various
specific impairments that interfere with response. These realities
create significant problems when employing traditional evaluation
methodologies that require the use of standardized tests, control
groups, and random assignment to treatment groups.

The *medically at-risk* population presents somewhat different
problems. *First,* great diversity exists in the selection of parameters
for defining this population (Ramey, Zeskind & Hunter, 1981).
Newborn Intensive Care Units often employ considerably different
criteria for assignment of the at-risk label to an infant. *Second,* care
for these infants may differ dramatically. For example, an infant
who is born in a rural area and experiences difficulties may have to
be transported to the nearest major medical center for care versus an
infant who is born in the center and receives highly specialized care
immediately. *Third,* many of the medically at-risk population appear to recover without any formal intervention. A most perplexing difficulty is the field's current inability to predict who of the
medically at-risk population will recover and who will not (Sigman,
Cohen & Forsythe, 1981). Some of the infants who appear to be
most distressed during the prenatal period recover without problem while others who appear less impaired do not recover and over
time show more serious disabilities such as cerebral palsy (Taft,
1981).

## Instrument Problems

A second problem that interferes with evaluating the impact of early intervention is the availability of appropriate instruments or measures. A large number of assessment instruments for infants exists (Cross & Johnston, 1977) but the majority of these instruments were developed for use with nonhandicapped children. Although many instruments were designed to assist in the identification and diagnosis of early childhood problems, developers rarely intended that these measures be employed to assess program impact.

Limitations of norm-referenced tests have led to the development of criterion-referenced and home-made measures. Unfortunately the majority of these instruments are not widely used and therefore adequate subject pools have not been generated to permit the development of expectancies or norms for subpopulations of handicapped or at-risk infants. In addition, these instruments are not used with sufficient numbers of subjects to collect adequate reliability and validity data.

## Design Problems

Traditional or even quasi-experimental research designs are often impossible to implement with populations of *handicapped* infants. Due to small heterogeneous groups and ethical considerations, random or matched assignment to control groups are not options (Bricker, Sheehan & Littman, 1981; Sheehan & Gallagher, 1983). Often the use of comparison or contrast groups is fraught with difficulties as well (Bricker & Sheehan, 1981). Most often intervention researchers are forced to adopt pre-post or retrospective comparisons (Simeonsson, Cooper & Scheiner, 1982) which are open to familiar and legitimate criticism.

The use of traditional designs with groups of *medically at-risk* populations can be undertaken with less difficulty for several reasons. *First,* there are generally larger groups of these infants available for study. *Second,* they do not have specific biological impairments, thus matching becomes less difficult. *Third,* there appear to be fewer ethical concerns about assignment of these infants to control groups or procedures. *Finally,* a selection bias may be operating in terms of those parents who either choose to participate in a study or to maintain once a study is begun (Cornell & Gottfried, 1976). The less interested parent may choose not to become involved or lose interest. For example, Scarr-Salapatek and Williams (1973) reported that all the experimental infants/parents maintained in the program and were available for follow-up while in the control group, five parents (over 30% of the sample) discontinued their participation and thus were unavailable for follow-up. It is difficult to determine how the results of this study might have differed if these infants had remained in the control group.

### Dependent and Independent Variables

Another problem facing evaluators of early intervention programs is the match between the *dependent and independent variables.* The dependent measure should reflect the program's emphasis, however often there is a mismatch between the program emphasis and the content of the measure selected to assess the impact of the intervention. Should a program that focuses on enhancement of the caregiver-infant interactions and social-communicative behavior use a measure of general cognitive functioning to assess program impact? For example, Rynders and Horrobin (1980) report the use of evaluation procedures that reflected the emphasis of their program and procedures that measured general growth. Interestingly they report that the experimental group failed to show significant differences on the program-relevant measures but did show significant differences on the more general cognitive measure. They concluded the program was ineffective, but is this the only feasible conclusion? In a study conducted by Harris (1981) an opposite effect was reported. That is, the Down's syndrome infants who participated in a short-term therapeutic intervention program showed significant growth in program specific objectives but did not show similar change on a more general standardized measure. Should one conclude that this program was effective or ineffective?

### Cost

A final constraint to be reckoned with when evaluating the effectiveness of early intervention programs is the *cost* involved. Most early intervention programs do not have the financial resources necessary to conduct systematic research on the impact of the program in ways that would be acceptable to the scientific community. The cost of longitudinal tracking of sizable groups of children is staggering and most agencies are unable to support such efforts. Further, changes that occur over spans of years are often significant and measuring the impact of such change is complicated because of change occurring in other areas.

The constraints discussed above are not offered as an apology but rather to alert the reader to the realities that face the intervention researcher. The outcomes of early intervention programs with handicapped and medically at-risk infants can be more fairly judged in the light of these constraints.

## INTERVENTION OUTCOMES
## WITH HANDICAPPED INFANTS

### Population Description

Data on the precise number of handicapped infants are difficult to obtain except for those infants who have clearly identifiable handicaps at birth, such as hydrocephalus (Hayden & Beck, 1983). Subgroups of handicapped infants that can be identified shortly after birth include those with genetic disorders such as Down's syndrome or central nervous system (CNS) abnormalities such as spina bifida. Hayden and Beck (1983) have assembled information that suggests approximately 160 infants per 100,000 have a serious genetic or CNS defect. Infants whose handicaps are less severe or who do not have an obvious physical manifestation are more difficult to identify during the first year. Later these babies attract attention when they either fail or are significantly delayed in attainment of expected developmental milestones (e.g., crawling, walking, talking).

The wide range of disabilities seen in infants and the differences when problems become manifest or are detected require that infant intervention programs often serve babies from birth to 36 months who display considerable variability in their behavioral repertoires. Depending upon the population base, some locales are able to offer programs for selected sub-groups of handicapped infants. For example, a number of programs have been developed exclusively for Down's syndrome babies (Hayden & Haring, 1977; Clunies-Ross, 1979). Smaller Towns and rural areas may offer programs that include infants from birth to 36 months with a variety of etiologies and who have a range of disabilities (Bricker & Sheehan, 1981). Most early intervention programs for handicapped infants serve a highly diverse population even if some specific criteria are used to select participants.

## Program Descriptions

According to Filler (1983) there are three major service delivery models used by early intervention programs: *home-based, center-based* and a *combination of home- and center-based.* Often programs for infants deliver services in the home. The target is the parent or caregiver who is helped to acquire intervention skills to use with the child. For example, Hanson and Schwarz (1978) have described a *home-based model* for Down's syndrome infants that they report produces significant growth in the participating infants.

As implied in the name, the *center-based model* requires that the infant be brought to an educational setting on a regular basis. The setting might be a classroom or a more informal arrangement. The focal target in center-based models is usually the infant; however, many center-based programs stress parental involvement (Rynders & Horrobin, 1980; Bricker & Sheehan, 1981) and may even provide structured training for the parent.

Some programs have adopted a *combined approach* in one of two ways. First, there are programs that stress training in the classroom and in the home (Hayden & Haring, 1977). Second, there are programs for the handicapped infant that initially employ a home-based model, and after the child reaches a certain age or develops targeted skills, transfers to the center-based component of the program (Kysela, Hillyard, McDonald & Ahlsten-Taylor, 1981).

Although a range of service delivery models is possible, in most locales, except for large metropolitan areas, program options are unavailable to families/children. A singular approach may be advisable from the perspective of funding and administration but often the lack of flexibility in service delivery results in the families/children making all the adjustments. Thus, local, state and federal agencies charged with providing services to handicapped infants need to begin to explore legislative, funding and administrative options that would permit interventionists more flexibility in the manner in which services became available to infants and their families.

*Two interesting shifts in programs have occurred recently. First,* programs are making concerted efforts to include the parent/family as integral members of the intervention team. Parent involvement has been a major issue during the 70s and the resolution appears to be that successful intervention with infants is highly dependent upon the program's ability to involve the parent/family. A *second* issue that currently permeates the literature on early intervention is the need to refocus instructional content to be maximally relevant for the infant/child. That is, instructional objectives should be chosen that are relevant and functional for individual children rather than being selected for a priori reasons.

The majority of programs providing services to handicapped infants tend to offer a comprehensive menu of educational objects. The comprehensive nature of the programs is appropriate because handicapped infants tend to show deficits in many critical areas of functioning. There is often need to assist the infant in gaining skills in cognitive, communication, social, self-help and motor areas.

Instructional approaches and content for early intervention programs are distributed across a continuum from direct instruction in which the infant is given little choice in the nature of the instructional program or the form of the response to those with an experiential emphasis in which the infant is free to choose from a variety of options throughout the instructional day. Harbin (1979) has suggested that current curricular foci can be classified as: *experiential, Montessori, Piagetian, information processing, diagnostic-perspective* or *behavioral.* As one moves away from the experiential end of the continuum the approach becomes increasingly teacher directed.

In programs that adopt a behavioral approach much of the instruction is provided during individual structured training sessions. The teacher selects the activities and the schedule for their presentation. More experiential oriented programs tend to provide the infants with less direct instruction. Rather, the children are offered more freedom to select and engage in activities. In actuality, most programs appear to adopt features of many curricular approaches so that one sees infants exposed to a variety of materials, instructional formats and activities.

### *Effectiveness of Early Intervention With Handicapped Infants*

Descriptions of intervention efforts with handicapped infants are plentiful yet many fail to provide any objective data that evaluate the effectiveness or impact of the program on the enrolled infants and their families. However, a core group of investigations exists that does provide various types of evaluative data and thus is a source for drawing some conclusions about program effectiveness (see Bricker, Bailey & Bruder, in press; Dunst & Rheingrover, 1981; Simeonsson, Cooper & Scheiner, 1982; Odom & Fewell, 1983).

When reviewing the early intervention efficacy data for handicapped infants several issues confront the reviewer/evaluator. Of primary concern is the variability found in the population served and the *duration, intensity* and *focus* of the program. In reviewing the 27 studies included in their analysis of early intervention programs for handicapped infants, Simeonsson, Cooper and Scheiner (1982) found that:

> Treatment group size ranged from 2 to 75 subjects, and age of subjects ranged from 2 1/2 months to more than 6 years. The reported frequency of sessions ranged from daily sessions to two occasions per week. Duration of individual sessions ranged from as brief as five minutes to as long as a full morning. The duration of the total early intervention programs ranged from a short four weeks to two years. (p. 636)

Such ranges in services and programs require considerable caution when drawing general conclusions about the effectiveness of early intervention.

In spite of the many problems facing those interested in examining the impact of early intervention with handicapped infants, a surprising number of reviewers have concluded that *early intervention with handicapped infants is effective.* The Simeonsson et al. (1982) analysis found that "48% of the studies reviewed yielded statistical evidence for effectiveness . . . " However, they noted that 93% of the studies reported effectiveness. Simeonsson et al. (1982) suggest the discrepancy between the 48% and 93% figures may be because the: (1) infants made progress but limited sample sizes precluded statistically significant gains, (2) infants made progress in areas not measured by the dependent measures, and (3) infants made no progress but change occurred in the parents or family.

Bricker, Bailey and Bruder (in press) reviewed a number of efficacy studies conducted with handicapped infants. The majority of these studies, albeit methodologically flawed, consistently reported significant child change on the dependent measures. In addition, a few studies reported positive outcomes for parents or families. Finally, Bricker et al. (in press) assembled data from several sources that suggest early intervention is cost effective.

In addition to general reviews of early intervention programs, some limited data are available on children with specific disabilities. Fraiberg and her colleagues (Adelson & Fraiberg, 1975) have reported the positive impact of early intervention on a small group of blind infants. Horton (1976) has reported similar findings for hearing impaired children. Molnar (1983), Harris (1981) and Soboloff (1981) have presented data that suggest physically handicapped infants and their parents can benefit from certain forms of therapeutic and educational intervention.

While one can find antagonists to the conclusion that early intervention with handicapped infants is effective (see Ferry, 1981; Piper & Pless, 1980; Gibson & Fields, in press), as Stedman notes (1983):

> In the final analysis, even given the cautions, design problems and difficulties with data interpretation, we already know a great deal about the effectiveness of (early) educational intervention. Generally the effects are positive. (p. 269)

A few examples of positive outcomes reported in the literature will emphasize Stedman's conclusion.

Several investigations that have focused on measuring early programming impact on the handicapped infants report significant gains on standardized measures such as the Bayley (Bricker & Sheehan, 1981), the Griffiths (Aronson & Fallstrom, 1977) and the Binet (Rynders & Horrobin, 1980). Other investigators have reported significant gains when using more programmatic measures. For example, Harris (1981) reports reliable gains on physical therapy treatment objectives for an experimental group of Down's syndrome infants. Kysela et al. (1981) indicate infants enrolled in an early intervention program showed significant progress towards the acquisition of functional language skills. In addition to gains reported for the infants, some programs also have attempted to examine effects on parents. A number of programs have demonstrated that parents can acquire instructional skills that impact their infant's performance (Baker & Heifetz, 1976; Filler & Kasari, 1981; Johnson, 1975).

The investigations cited above highlight the available literature on program impact. Taken in the context of the methodological constraints inherent in intervention research, a general conclusion seems warranted. *Early intervention appears to assist infants in maximizing their independent functioning and their families in obtaining knowledge and skills that enhance their adjustment to the infant.*

## INTERVENTION OUTCOMES
## WITH MEDICALLY AT-RISK INFANTS

### Population Description

The majority of infants classified as medically at-risk are born prematurely and/or have a low birth weight because length of gestation and weight are highly correlated. Eighty-five percent of births occur within the normal range for gestation and birth weight leaving 15% that are either premature or low-birth weight or both (Keller, 1981). Prematurity or low-birth weight, unless extreme, do not of themselves produce problems. Rather, it is the associated conditions that cause problems (e.g., respiratory problems, or regulation of body temperature). In addition to premature birth, other conditions can result in assigning the label medically at-risk to infants. These conditions can include toxemia, asphyxia, infection or respiratory problems (Werthmann, 1981) to mention a few.

The array of problems represented in the medically at-risk population results in substantial variations in the infants who compose this group, although it is short of the extreme heterogeneity found in populations of handicapped infants. A further problem arises for the interventionist, however, in that the majority of medically at-risk infants recover completely without any form of formal intervention. Approximately 30% of the infants discharged from Neonatal Intensive Care Units will require some form of intervention by age 6 (Scott & Masi, 1979). This suggests that 70% of the youngsters will have the necessary self-righting tendencies to recover from an early insult such as low-birth weight or prematurity. Also, as mentioned above, investigators have not yet found any medical indices that are adequate predictors of the infants' subsequent outcomes (McCall, 1979). Family educational level and income level continue to be the most accurate predictors of later outcomes for infants (Sameroff, 1981). Finally it should be emphasized that most of the intervention studies conducted with the medically at-risk population are focused on the *premature infant*.

### Program Description

Most medically at-risk infants require some form of medical intervention (such as mechanical ventilation, supplemental oxygen, drugs to control infection, surgery to repair structural defects and so forth). Once the infant has passed the acute or crisis stage during which the major concern is often survival, other forms of early intervention have been attempted. These formal interventions can be conveniently divided into those that attempt to assist the infant in regulation of the body and its processes and those that attempt to provide some form of stimulation that will enrich the infant's behavioral repertoire. The first type of intervention tends to occur prior to the infant's discharge from the NICU. These procedures primarily attempt to replace or remediate environmental deficiencies and thus can be thought of as compensatory approaches. The second type of intervention approach operates from the conceptual position that at-risk infants will benefit from extra stimulation.

Compensatory approaches often tend to try to simulate conditions the infant experiences in the womb. The rationale is that the premature infant entered the world before he/she was ready and thus attempts are made to recapture beneficial aspects of the fetal environment. An array of strategies have been undertaken; for example, piping heart beats into the infant's isolette, rocking the infant, or increased handling or touching of the infant.

Extra-stimulation programs offer a different approach in that the infant is provided some systematic presentation of an activity or stimulation that might not otherwise occur. A frequent approach has been to provide the parent with information and/or training designed to enhance their interaction with the infant. For example, the UCLA Infant Studies Project (Bromwich & Parmelee, 1979) provided systematic assistance to families in the home setting. A home-visitor attempted to share information and suggest activities that were designed to enhance the parental enjoyment of, and sensitivity to, their infant. Minde and his colleagues (Minde, Shosenberg, Marton, Thompson, Ripley, & Burns, 1980) offered parents who had infants in the NICU the opportunity to participate in weekly discussion groups. Another extra-stimulation strategy has been to train professional staff to provide specific interventions with infants (Barnard, 1976). Leib, Benfield and Guidubaldi (1980) had the NICU staff hang mobiles in the infants' isolettes, provide extra tactile stimulation during feeding, and play music boxes for the infants.

## EFFECTIVENESS OF EARLY INTERVENTION WITH MEDICALLY AT-RISK INFANTS

A major difference between the intervention studies undertaken with populations of handicapped infants and premature infants is that studies of intervention efforts with the premature infant generally report the inclusion of a non-intervention control. Many studies randomly assigned infants to experimental or control groups and thus were able to examine the impact of the intervention procedure more objectively. Even so, Cornell and Gottfried (1976) report that many of these studies had methodological problems which render their outcomes somewhat suspect.

For the most part the reported outcomes for premature infants involving some form of compensatory or supplemental stimulation are positive (Masi, 1979). The infants receiving the experimental treatment generally perform significantly better than the controls on the selected dependent measure. However, this finding requires cautious interpretation for two reasons. First, the dependent measures selected tend to vary considerably (e.g., weight gain, amount of crying, IQ scores), thus little consistency of effect is reportable. Second, when a consistent dependent measure is found, the reported outcomes vary. For example, Cornell and Gottfried (1976) found that of the 9 studies they examined that used weight gain, 5 reported no difference while 4 reported differences. Nevertheless, a number of researchers and clinicians support early intervention efforts and are comfortable in concluding that the procedures tried have generally produced positive impacts on infants and families (Masi, 1979; Bromwich & Parmelee, 1979; Taft, 1981).

A final concern noted about early intervention efforts with at-risk infants is the often weak conceptual foundation used to develop compensatory or supplemental procedures (Keogh & Kopp, 1978). In particular, both Ramey, Zeskind and Hunter (1981) and Fagan and Singer (1981) question the usefulness of general stimulation models. Rather these investigators argue for the development of models which provide *specificity for determining the infant's deficit and specificity for selection of remedial procedures to eliminate the identified problem.*

It is important to remember that attempts to enhance the development of the premature infant are new. The data and information generated during the past 20 years provide a rich foundation for developing more adequate models and effective procedures.

## GENERAL SUMMARY

The purpose of this article has been to discuss the impact of early intervention programs on handicapped and medically at-risk infants. The approaches that have been adopted to provide educational and therapeutic services to handicapped and at-risk infants share some commonalities as well as differences. *The uniformity* is most apparent in the programs' universal attempt to assist infants directly or indirectly to compensate for absent or deficient behaviors. *The differences* emerge as one compares the instructional content and approach adopted to assist the infant and/or parent in reaching established goals. When these different intervention approaches have been studied, and/or compared with no treatment, the results are overwhelmingly positive. Investigators have consistently reported significant progress for infants and in many cases for parents. Although careful analysis of this data base has uncovered flaws, reviewers uniformly suggest that efforts be continued to devise thoughtful and effective interventions for distressed infants. Few investigators have suggested that efforts to devise therapeutic routines and environments for these infants be abandoned. The accumulation of more objective outcomes documenting the impact of early intervention is needed, but it is important to note the recency of the venture, the progress to date, and the considerable optimism expressed by interventionists for the future.

## REFERENCES

Adelson, E., & Fraiberg, S. (1975). Gross motor development in infants blind from birth. In B. Friedlander, G. Sterritt, & G. Kirk (Eds.), *Exceptional infant: Vol. 3*. New York: Brunner/Mazel.

Aronson, M., & Fallstrom, K. Immediate and long-term effects of developmental training in children with Down's syndrome. *Developmental Medicine and Child Neurology, 19*, 489-494.

Baker, B., & Heifetz, L., (1976). The Read Project: Teaching manuals for parents of retarded children. In T. Tjossem (Ed.), *Intervention strategies for high risk infants and young children*. Baltimore: University Park Press.

Barnard, K. (1976). Nursing: High risk infants. In T. Tjossem (Ed.), *Intervention strategies for high risk infants and young children*. Baltimore, MD: University Park Press.

Bricker, D., Bailey, E., & Bruder, M. (in press). The efficacy of early intervention and the handicapped infant: A wise or wasted resource? *Advances in Developmental and Behavioral Pediatrics, Vol. V*.

Bricker, D., & Sheehan, R. (1981). Effectiveness of an early intervention program as indexed by child change. *Journal of the Division for Early Childhood, 4*, 11-27.

Bricker, D., Sheehan, R., & Littman, D. (1981). Early intervention: A plan for evaluating program impact. WESTAR Publication, Seattle, WA.

Bromwich, R., & Parmelee, A. (1979). An intervention program for pre-term infants. In T. Field, A. Sostek, S. Goldberg, & H. Shuman (Eds.), *Infants born at risk*. Jamaica, NY: Spectrum Publications.

Clunies-Ross, G. (1979). Accelerating the development of Down's syndrome infants and young children. *The Journal of Special Education, 13*, 169-177.

Cornell, E., & Gottfried, A. (1976). Intervention with premature human infants. *Child Development, 47*, 32-39.

Cross, L., & Johnston, S. (1977). A bibliography of instruments. In L. Cross & K. Goin (Eds.), *Identifying handicapped children: A guide to casefinding, screening, diagnosis, assessment, and evaluation.* New York: Walker Publishing Co.

Dunst, C., & Rheingrover, R. (1981). An analysis of the efficacy of infant intervention program with organically handicapped children. *Evaluation and Program Planning, 4,* 287-323.

Fagan, J., & Singer, L. (1981). Intervention during infancy: General considerations. In S. Friedman & M. Sigman (Eds.), *Preterm birth and psychological development.* New York: Academic Press.

Ferry, P. (1981). On growing new neurons: Are early intervention programs effective? *Pediatrics, 67,* 38-41.

Filler, J. (1983). Service models for handicapped infants. In G. Garwood & R. Fewell (Eds.), *Educating handicapped infants.* Rockville, MD: An Aspen Publication.

Filler, J., & Kasari, C. (1981). Acquisition, maintenance and generalization of parent-taught skills with two severely handicapped infants. *The Journal of the Association for the Severely Handicapped, 6,* 30-38.

Garwood, G. (1982). Early childhood intervention: Is it time to change outcome variables? *Topics in Early Childhood Special Education, 1,* ix-xi.

Gibson, D., & Fields, D. (in press). Early stimulation programs for Down's syndrome: An effectiveness inventory. In M. Wolraich (Ed.), *Advances in Behavioral and Developmental Pediatrics, Vol. 5.* Greenwich, Conn.: JAI Press.

Hanson, M., & Schwarz, R. (1978). Results of a longitudinal intervention program for Down's syndrome infants and their families. *Education and Training of the Mentally Retarded, 13,* 403-407.

Harbin, G. (1979). Mildly to moderately handicapped preschoolers: How do you select child assessment instruments? In T. Black (Ed.), *Perspectives on measurement: A collection of readings for educators of young handicapped children.* Chapel Hill, NC: TADS.

Harris, S. (1981). Effects of neurodevelopmental therapy on motor performance of infants with Down's syndrome. *Developmental Medicine and Child Neurology, 23,* 477-483.

Hayden, A., & Beck, G. (1982). The epidemiology of high-risk and handicapped infants. In C. Ramey & P. Trohanis (Eds.), *Finding and educating high-risk and handicapped infants.* Baltimore, MD: University Park Press.

Hayden, A., & Haring, N. (1977). The acceleration and maintenance of developmental gains in Down's syndrome school-age children. In P. Mittler (Ed.), *Research to practice in mental retardation. Volume I Care and Intervention.* Baltimore: University Park Press.

Horton, K. (1976). Early intervention for hearing-impaired infants and young children. In T. Tjossem (Ed.), *Intervention strategies for high risk infants and young children.* Baltimore, MD: University Park Press.

Johnson, D. (1975). The development of a program for parent-child education among Mexican-Americans in Texas. In B. Friedlander, G. Sterritt, & G. Kirk (Eds.), *Exceptional infant: Assessment and intervention, Vol. 3.* New York: Brunner/Mazel.

Keller, C. (1981). Epidemiological characteristics of preterm births. In S. Friedman & M. Sigman (Eds.), *Preterm birth and psychological development.* New York: Academic Press.

Keogh, B., & Kopp, C. (1978). From assessment to intervention: An elusive bridge. In F. Minifie & Lloyd (Eds.), *Communicative and cognitive abilities—early behavioral assessment.* Baltimore, MD: University Park Press.

Kysela, G., Hillyard, A., McDonald, L., & Taylor, J. (1981). Early intervention, design and evaluation. In R. Schiefelbusch & D. Bricker (Eds.), *Early language: Acquisition and intervention.* Baltimore: University Park Press.

Leib, S., Benfield, G., & Guidubaldi, J. (1980). Effects of early intervention and stimulation on the preterm infant. *Pediatrics, 66,* 83-90.

Masi, W. (1979). Supplemental stimulation of the premature infant. In T. Field (Ed.), *Infants born at risk.* New York: Spectrum.

McCall, R. (1979). The development of intellectual functioning in infancy and the prediction of later IQ. In J. Osofsky (Ed.), *Handbook of infant development.* New York: Wiley.

Minde, K., Shosenberg, N., Marton, P., Thompson, J., Ripley, J., & Burns, S. (1980). Self help groups in a premature nursery—A controlled evaluation. *The Journal of Pediatrics, 96,* 933-940.

Molnar, G. (1982). Intervention for physically handicapped children. In M. Lewis & L. Taft (Eds.), *Developmental disabilities theory, assessment and intervention.* New York: Spectrum.

Odom, S., & Fewell, R. (1983). Program evaluation in early childhood special education: A meta-evaluation. *Educational Evaluation and Policy Analysis, 5,* 445-460.

Piper, M., & Pless, I. (1980). Early intervention for infants with Down's syndrome: A controlled trial. *Pediatrics, 65,* 463-468.

Ramey, C., Zeskind, P., & Hunter, R. (1981). Biomedical and psychosocial intervention for preterm infants. In S. Friedman & M. Sigman (Eds.), *Preterm birth and psychological development.* New York: Academic Press.

Rynders, J., & Horrobin, M. (1980). Educational provisions for young children with Down's syndrome. In J. Gottlieb (Ed.), *Educating mentally retarded persons in the mainstream.* Baltimore, MD: University Park Press.

Sameroff, A. (1981). Longitudinal studies of preterm infants: A review of chapters 17-20. In S. Friedman & M. Sigman (Eds.), *Preterm birth and psychological development.* New York: Academic Press.

Scarr-Salapatek, S., & Williams, M. (1973). The effects of early stimulation on low-birth-weight infants. *Child Development. 44,* 94-101.

Scott, K., & Masi, W. (1979). The outcome from the utility of registers of risk. In T. Field, A. Sostek, S. Goldberg, & H. Shuman (Eds.), *Infants born at risk.* Jamaica, NY: Spectrum Publications.

Sheehan, R., & Gallagher, R. (1983). Conducting evaluations of infant intervention. In G. Garwood & R. Fewell (Eds.), *Educating handicapped infants.* Rockville, MD: Aspen Publications.

Sigman, M., Cohen, S., & Forsythe, A. (1981). The relation of early infant measures to later development. In S. Friedman & M. Sigman (Eds.), *Preterm birth and psychological development.* New York: Academic Press.

Simeonsson, R., Cooper, D., & Scheiner, A. (1982). A review and analysis of the effectiveness of early intervention programs. *Pediatrics, 69,* 635-641.

Soboloff, H. (1981). Early intervention—Fact or fiction? *Developmental Medicine and Child Neurology, 23,* 261-266.

Stedman, D. (1982). The effect of educational intervention programs on the cognitive development of young children. In M. Lewis & L. Taft (Eds.), *Developmental disabilities theory, assessment and intervention.* New York: Spectrum.

Taft, L. (1981). Intervention programs for infants with cerebral palsy: A clinician's view. In C. Brown (Ed.), *Infants at risk.* Johnson & Johnson Baby Products Company Pediatric Round Table Series, 5.

Werthmann, M. (1981). Medical constraints to optimal psychological development of the preterm infant. In S. Friedman & M. Sigman (Eds.), *Preterm birth and psychological development.* New York: Academic Press.

# Intervention Programs
# for Adolescent Mothers
# and Their Offspring

Susan C. McDonough, PhD

**ABSTRACT.** Interest in the problems associated with adolescent childbearing and childrearing has stimulated numerous efforts at primary and secondary prevention of teenage pregnancy and a plethora of programs designed to minimize the problems faced by an adolescent mother in rearing a child. Although the specific goals of a given intervention program for adolescent mothers and their offspring may vary, most programs focus on eliminating or minimizing the deleterious consequences of early childbearing and childrearing. Programs were reviewed according to commonly cited intervention goals. Although each program reported moderate success with a particular intervention approach, the research to date is insufficient to recommend one intervention strategy over another.

Over the past twenty years the incidence of out-of-wedlock pregnancies has increased rapidly. An estimated 10% of U.S. adolescents become pregnant annually. Although birthrates among every maternal age group in the country are declining, among teenagers the decline is only apparent among older adolescents. Out-of-wedlock pregnancy has increased by 75% among adolescents 17 years of age or younger. Approximately 600,000 live births per year result from these pregnancies in this age group (Alan Guttmacher Institute, 1976).

## CONSEQUENCES OF ADOLESCENT CHILDBEARING

For adolescents, premature motherhood often means an interruption in their own education and subsequent lack of vocational

Susan C. McDonough is Director of Training and Research Scientist at the Institute for the Study of Developmental Disabilities, University of Illinois at Chicago, 1640 W. Roosevelt Road, Chicago, IL 60608.

training. Economic dependency, poverty, larger family size, and social isolation are factors associated with adolescent childbearing (Card, 1981; Finkelstein, Finkelstein, Christie, Roden, & Skelton, 1982; Gunter & La Barba, 1981; Phipps-Yonas, 1980; Seitz, Apfel, & Rosenbaum, 1983). These consequences of early pregnancy and motherhood are not limited only to the adolescent mother and her offspring. The birth of an infant to a teenager usually means increased psychological and financial burdens on the adolescent's own family. The teenager's parents find themselves in a position of making room for another child during a period in their own adult lives when they expected to be free from the responsibilities of child rearing (Smith, 1975). Also, the adolescent mother's failure to achieve her educational goals and to acquire vocational skills represents a significant cost to society both in the loss of human potential and the expenses associated with the provision of services (Peabody, McKenry & Corders, 1981). The cost of potentially life-long support of these unskilled mothers and their offspring has yet to be determined.

Interest in the problems associated with adolescent childbearing and childrearing has stimulated numerous efforts at primary and secondary prevention of teenage pregnancy and a plethora of programs designed to minimize the problems faced by an adolescent mother in rearing a child (Badger, Burns, Rhoads, 1976; Bennett & Bardon, 1977; Cartoof, 1978; Field, Widmayer, Stringer, & Ignatoff, 1980; Lyon, 1979; McDonough, 1984; Nelson, Key, Fletcher, Kirpatrick, & Feinstein, 1982; Olds, 1983; Schneider, 1982). Individuals differ in their opinions of what constitutes effective intervention strategies. Who should be targeted for such interventions and when is intervention optimal: before conception, before birth, or after birth? However, everyone appears to agree that prevention of out-of-wedlock adolescent pregnancy and support for young mothers and their offspring is of paramount importance (Cobliner, 1981a; Jekel, 1981; McKenry, Walters, & Johnson, 1979; Phipps-Yonas, 1980).

## INTERVENTION PROGRAMS

The literature on intervention programs for teenage mothers and their offspring shares many of the same problems often faced in studies reporting on intervention results in the human services.

These potential difficulties include: adequacy and availability of control groups, choice of appropriate criteria to measure intervention effectiveness, and generalizability from one sample to another. In addition, many intervention reports tend to be descriptive, advocatory, and lack a strong theoretical focus. Consequently, in some of the adolescent mother literature it is difficult to tease apart the variables that account for the purported positive effects of a given intervention program. Are the perceived or documented positive effects the result of a specific intervention or can these positive outcomes be explained by an alternative hypothesis such as the emerging maturation and developing competence of the adolescent mother? With these qualifiers in mind we will review some of the various interventions dealing with teenage parents and their offspring currently reported in the literature.

Although the specific goals of a given intervention program for adolescent mothers and their offspring may vary, most programs focus on eliminating or minimizing the deleterious consequences of early childbearing and childrearing. In reviewing reports of program descriptions and objectives, four intervention goals repeatedly emerged:

1. Minimizing the obstetrical complications for the pregnant adolescent and the neonatal complications for the infant.
2. Fostering positive attitudes, parenting skills, and parent-child interactions.
3. Reducing the social isolation of the young mother and her infant.
4. Eliminating repeat out-of-wedlock pregnancies.

While the effect of intervention programs can be viewed from a variety of perspectives, the discussion will focus on the impact these programs have had on the lives of the clients they sought to serve. The programs are grouped and reviewed according to these commonly cited program goals.

## Minimizing Obstetrical and Neonatal Complications

The literature reports that adolescent mothers and their offspring appear to be at greater risk for physiological problems than older mothers (Finkelstein et al., 1982; Gunter & La Barba, 1981; Roosa, Fitzgerald, & Carson, 1982a, 1982b). According to several researchers, pregnant adolescents experienced higher rates of anemia, toxemia, hypertension, and prolonged labor (Baldwin & Cain, 1980; Gunter & La Barba, 1981). Children of teenage mothers appear to be at risk for prematurity, low birth weight, physical and neurological defects, and infant mortality (Alan Guttmacher Institute, 1976; McKenry et al., 1979). Other studies refute these claims.

In a Danish study of maternal age and complications in 9,125 births at an urban hospital, Mednick, Baker and Sutton-Smith (1979) report that adolescents experienced fewer complications during pregnancy than did older mothers. Sander and Vietze (1979) examined the relationship between maternal age and infant health in a sample from a Tennessee county hospital serving primarily low-income clients. The investigators found no differences between young and older mothers when quality of medical care was maintained. The participants in both the Mednick et al. (1979) and the Sander and Vietze (1979) studies were enrolled in high quality prenatal care programs early in their pregnancies. The critical variable in teenage childbearing may be the quality and quantity of the prenatal care available to the mother rather than the adolescent's physiological immaturity (Baldwin & Cain, 1980; Phipps-Yonas, 1980; Roosa et al., 1982a). As most teenage pregnancy occurs in low socioeconomic groups and social status has been shown to be related to the quality of obstetrical care available to the prospective mother, it seems reasonable to assume that the pregnant adolescent generally does not have access to high quality prenatal programs (Mednick et al., 1979).

Other studies support this interaction between the variables, particularly socioeconomic status. In a review of the effects economically deprived environments have on subsequent development, Birch and Gussow (1970) argued that high risk infant status is associated with low economic standing and ethnicity. The highest proportion of perinatal complications were found among populations which were poor and black. Investigators studying the way social status variables modulate the effects of perinatal factors report similar findings (Ramey, Collier, Sparling, Loda, Campbell, & Finkelstein, 1976; Heber & Garber, 1975; Sameroff & Chandler, 1975). These findings imply that the biological outcomes of pregnancy are worse for individuals in economically deprived areas regardless of maternal age.

## Fostering Positive Parental Attitudes, Parenting Skills and Parent-Child Interactions

The attachment literature has yielded much information concerning the relationship between infant cognitive and social development and attachment (Bell & Ainsworth, 1972). The importance of reciprocity and mutual satisfaction in the caregiver infant relationship is highlighted in studies which demonstrate the effect of the infant's behavior on that of the caregiver (Bromwich, 1976). These findings lend support to the current view that positive effect in caregiver infant interactions is a cornerstone of optimum infant development.

The ability of the mother to become attached to her infant and to engage in caretaking behavior is related to a complex of socioeconomic, educational, and personality factors (Sameroff, 1981). In order to focus on her infant, the mother must be able to separate her child's demands from her own needs. If a teenage mother is struggling with problems concerning her own self-identity (a common problem of adolescence), she likely will be unavailable to meet the needs of her infant. Sameroff's (1981) contention of emotional availability is supported by the majority of studies reported by Phipps-Yonas (1980) which suggest that teenage mothers are less emotionally available to their infants, engage in fewer verbal interactions, and offer less cognitive stimulation to their offspring. A notable exception is a report by Osofsky and Osofsky (1970) which offers a contrasting description of the adolescent mother's interactive behavior with her infant during routine, monthly pediatric visits. These adolescent mothers typically were observed displaying warmth and high amounts of physical interaction but little verbal communication with their infants. Their infants were rated as highly active but were evaluated as displaying little responsitivity to their mothers. These differing reports of mother infant interaction may be explained by other mediating factors such as maternal education, parenting attitudes, maternal childhood experience, knowledge of child development, personality factors, stress, or socioeconomic status among the sample of adolescent mothers studied.

Most prenatal intervention for pregnant adolescents include some information on the medical and nutritional needs of the newborn. To date, there are few reported studies of programs which have included information on child development and child rearing techniques. One exception is the Bennett and Bardon (1977) study which examined pregnant adolescents' knowledge of child development and behavior prior to the birth of their infants. The investigators found significant pre/posttest gains on the teenagers' knowledge of family life and human reproduction after having attended a comprehensive in-school program offering medical counseling and academic assistance.

In contrast to prenatal programs for adolescents, postnatal programs tend to focus on developing realistic attitudes regarding child behavior and development and on fostering good child care practices. This effort appears useful in light of the literature on adolescent parent childrearing attitudes and knowledge. In a study of adolescents' parental knowledge and skills in rural Pennsylvania, de Lissovoy (1973) found teenage parents to possess only limited factual knowledge on child development, to be insensitive to their infants' signals and needs, to be prone to use physical punishment, and to engage in little spontaneous cuddling. Smith, Mumford, and Hammer (1979) reporting on over 400 interviews of adolescent mothers, found similar results, especially for the very young teenager. Although the literature on this topic is sparse, investigators find that adolescent parents appear to lack the maternal attitudes, knowledge and abilities believed necessary for caregiving.

Data from postpartum intervention programs indicate that adolescent mothers can be trained to function more effectively as caregivers for their children. Field et al. (1980) reported that teenage mothers who were given a parent training intervention through biweekly home visits for four months engaged in more face-to-face interactions with their preterm infants and expressed more realistic childrearing attitudes and knowledge of child development than did a comparison group of mothers. Similarly, Badger et al. (1976) reported that adolescent mothers who took part in a postpartum child care program demonstrated increasingly more responsivity to the needs of their infants over the eight week intervention program.

In a less time consuming and costly intervention, Widmayer and Field (1980) found that teenage mothers of preterm infants who had observed a Brazelton demonstration during the neonatal period and who had completed weekly parent assessments of their infant's behavior interacted more positively with their infant at one month of age. The authors speculate that these positive effects may have been mediated by the young mothers' modeling of the infant examiner's response-eliciting behaviors observed during the Brazelton exam.

Reviewed in the aggregate, these studies and others (Garret,

1982; McDonough, 1984; Nelson et al., 1982; Osofsky & Osofsky, 1970) suggest that postpartum intervention can have a short-term, significantly positive impact on the attitudes, knowledge and inter-actional behavior of adolescent mothers. The long-term impact of these programs remains unclear.

## Reducing Social Isolation-Maximizing Support

Because early motherhood has consequences both for the adoles-cent and her offspring, intervention programs generally address the developmental, physical and psychological needs of the mother-infant dyad (Osofsky & Osofsky, 1970; Schneider, 1982; Wise & Grossman, 1980). Recently investigators have examined the effect of broadening the scope of intervention beyond this dyad to the so-cial and support system of the teenage mother and her child (Kel-lam, Adams, Brown, & Ensmenger, 1982; Olds, 1983; Smith, 1975). This expansion to other family members appears to be asso-ciated with a trend over the past decade for most young women who give birth out-of-wedlock to keep and rear their infants. Prior to this time many pregnant adolescents were living in residences separated from family and friends; few adolescent mothers decided to keep their babies (Alan Guttmacher Institute, 1976; Clapp & Raab, 1978; Seitz et al., 1983). Therefore, members of the pregnant adolescent's family were not involved with the professionals providing services to the young woman.

Today the unmarried pregnant adolescent who plans to keep her baby often remains in her family home throughout her pregnancy and after the birth of her child (Friedman, 1975; Held, 1981; Smith et al., 1979). Consequently, the adolescent's mother or grand-mother often is involved in the care of the infant (Smith, 1975). This is especially true in cases where the adolescent is interested and motivated to return to school and complete her education (Clapp & Raab, 1978). The need to work with the adolescent's family, espe-cially the teenager's own mother, seems to be critical for promoting family support for the adolescent and harmony around child rearing issues.

In a study examining self-esteem and social networks of 62 preg-nant adolescents from three ethnic groups, Black, White, and Mex-ican-American, Held (1981) found that adolescents from all three groups rated their mother as more important to themselves than they were. The social support perceived by the adolescents differed according to ethnic background. The mothers of Black teenagers appeared less likely to rate the pregnancy in a positive way but also were less likely to let it interrupt their daughters' education. Of the three ethnic groups, Mexican-American mothers seemed most approving of the pregnancy. Within their larger social network, 64% of the White adolescents perceived disapproval whereas Black teenagers perceived disapproval 43% of the time. Only 20% of the Mexican-American adolescents reported social disapproval from extended family and friends. It is important to note that unlike adolescents in the other groups, Mexican-American teenagers indicated a desire to marry and to have another child within the next two years.

This study refutes the persistent misconception that some minority families do not accept the pregnancy of an unmarried daughter. Often the family is angry and disappointed as they had hoped for a better life for their child than what they had been able to achieve (Smith, 1975). Even if disappointed and angry, the prospective grandmother (mother of the pregnant teenager) frequently assumes her parental role by providing guidance and consultation to her daughter around pregnancy issues, i.e., prenatal health care and delivery preparations. Although the pregnant adolescent is the appropriate focus of intervention program, providing a role for the teenager's mother in the intervention effort may foster the formation of a closer alliance between the pregnant daughter and her mother.

Until recently the teenage father usually has been overlooked as a potential participant in intervention programs. Reports of adolescent fathers currently in the literature tend to be studies of paternal characteristics (Elster & Panzarine, 1980; Nakashima & Camp, 1984) rather than the results of programmatic interventions which systematically included the father in treatment or counseling. As male adolescents are known to be more sexually active than female adolescents, and are sexually active at an earlier age (Alan Guttmacher Institute, 1976), it is important to involve both adolescent males and females in preparenthood, antepartum and postpartum intervention programs.

## Eliminating Repeat Out-of-Wedlock Pregnancies

Studies consistently have demonstrated that women who have their first child during their early teenage years tend to bear more children than women who postpone childbearing until 20 years of age. Investigators have found little support for the contention that contraceptive information and devices alone will eliminate repeat out-of-wedlock pregnancies (Cobbiner, 1981b; Lindeman & Scott, 1981; Peabody et al., 1981; Wise & Grossman, 1980). The major reasons cited by adolescents for non-use of contraception when it is available is the belief that pregnancy will not occur and that intercourse is unexpected. Lindermann and Scott (1981) contend that the quality of contraception information and the effectiveness of its implementation is relevant only if the teenager seeks to avoid pregnancy. These investigators argue that the pregnancies of many adolescents are not "unwanted". On the contrary, many young teenagers *want* to get pregnant.

In our society, as well as in most other societies, motherhood carries with it a positive value which leads unmarried adolescents to choose it in spite of the hardships and difficulties that were documented earlier. To a young person whose own future is bleak or uncertain, having a baby may not be the most desirable option, but it is a readily available one.

Adolescents' motives for becoming pregnant and having a baby can vary widely. They may be motivated by the excitement of a new experience, the desire to prove their fertility, and/or the wish to strengthen a relationship. Often teenage mothers express the desire to have someone to love and someone to love them. Knowing what motivates adolescents to choose early pregnancy and motherhood may provide us with the necessary information to create programs that are effective in preventing adolescent pregnancy rather than programs that are designed to deal solely with its consequences.

One finding that emerges from the literature is the trans-generational cycle of premature parenting. In a longitudinal study of mothers in three boroughs of New York City, Presser (1980) assessed the consequences of a woman having a first birth during her adolescence versus having a first child in her twenties. Presser found the best predictor of a young woman's first birth was the age at which her own mother had given birth. A study by Card (1981) reported similar results in a 15 year follow-up of participants from Project TALENT, a national longitudinal survey of 375,000 teenagers who were in grades 9 to 12 in 1960.

The offspring of women who gave birth as adolescents themselves or the younger sisters of pregnant teenagers or adolescent mothers may be a target group with whom to work for the prevention of future teenage pregnancies. The younger the adolescent the greater the risk of pregnancy because contraceptives are used less by younger teenagers. Consequently, intervention efforts should be directed at reaching adolescents prior to the time they become sexually active.

## CONCLUSION

Programs espousing a variety of intervention goals and intervention strategies have been reviewed in the paper. Although each program reported moderate success with a particular intervention approach, the research to date is insufficient to recommend one intervention strategy over another. It does seem clear that our society must offer options *other than premature parenthood* to adolescents that enhance their self-esteem, feelings of self-worth, and that encourage teenagers to engage in the more appropriate developmental tasks of adolescence.

## REFERENCES

Alan Guttmacher Institute. 1976. *11 Million teenagers: What can be done about the epidemic of adolescent pregnancies in the United States.* New York: Planned Parenthood of America, 1976.

Badger, E., Burns, D., & Rhoads, B. 1976. Education for adolescent mothers in a hospital setting. *American Journal of Public Health, 66,* 469-472.

Baldwin, W. & Cain, V.S. 1980. The children of teenage parents. *Family Planning Perspectives, 12*(1), 34-43.

Bell, S.M., & Ainsworth, M.D.S. 1972. Infant crying and maternal responsiveness. *Child Development, 43,* 1171-1190.

Bennett, V. & Bardon, J.I. 1977. The effects of a school program on teenage mothers and their children. *American Journal of Orthopsychiatry, 47,* 671-678.

Birch, H., & Gussow, G.D. 1970. *Disadvantaged Children.* New York: Grune & Stratton.

Bromwich, R.M. 1976. Focus on maternal behavior in infant intervention. *American Journal of Orthopsychiatry, 46*(3), 439-446.

Card, J.J. 1981. Long-term consequences for children of teenage parents. *Demography, 18*(2), 137-156.

Cartoof, V. 1978. Postpartum services for adolescent mothers. *Child Welfare, 57,* 600-666.

Clapp, D.F. & Raab, R.S. 1978. Follow-up of unmarried adolescent mothers. *Social Work, 22,* 149-153.

Cobliner, W.H. 1981a. Prevention of adolescent pregnancy: A developmental perspective. In E.R. McAnarney and G. Stickle (Eds.), *Pregnancy and childbearing during adolescence: Research priorities for the 1980's.* New York: Alan R. Liss, Inc., p. 35-48.

Cobliner, W.G. 1981b. Who is most at risk? *The Female Patient, 6,* 63-68.

deLissovoy, V. 1973. Child care by adolescent parents. *Children Today, 2*(4), 22-25.

Elster, A.B. & Panzarine, S. 1980. Unwed teenage fathers. *Journal of Adolescent Health Care, 1,* 116-120.

Field, T.M., Widmayer, S., Stringer, S., & Ignataff, E. 1980. An intervention and developmental follow-up of preterm infants born to teenage, lower class mothers. *Child Development, 51,* 426-436.

Finkelstein, F., Finkelstein, J.A., Christie, M., Roden, M., & Skelton, C. 1982. Teenage pregnancy and parenthood: Outcomes for mother and child. *Journal of Adolescent Health Care, 3,* 1-7.

Friedman, H.L. 1975. Why are they keeping their babies? *Social Work, 20,* 322-323.

Garret, C.J. 1982. Programs designed to respond to adolescent pregnancies. In N. Anastasiow. *The Adolescent Parent.* Baltimore: Paul H. Brookes Publishing Co., Inc. p. 67-82.

Gunter, N.C. & LaBarba, R.C. 1981. Maternal and perinatal effects of adolescent childbearing. *American Journal of Behavioral Development, 4*(3), 333-357.

Heber, R., & Garber, H. 1975. The Milwaukee Project: A study of the use of family intervention to prevent cultural-familial mental retardation. In B.Z. Friedlander, G.M. Sterritt, & G.E. Kirk (Eds.), In *Exceptional infant: Assessment and intervention.* New York: Brunner-Mazel, p. 399-433.

Held, L. 1981. Self-esteem and social network of the young pregnant teenager. *Adolescence, 16*(64), 905-912.

Jekel, J.F. 1981. Evaluations of programs of adolescents. In E. McAnarney and G. Stickle (Eds.), *Pregnancy and childbearing during adolescence: Research priorities for the 1980's.* New York: Alan R. Liss, Inc., p. 139-154.

Kellam, S.G., Adams, R.G., Brown, C.H., & Ensmenger, M.E. 1982. The long-term evaluation of the family structure of teenage and older mothers. *Journal of Marriage and the Family, 44,* 539-554.

Lindemann, C., & Scott, W.J. 1981. Wanted and unwanted pregnancy in early adolescence: Evidence from a clinic population. *Journal of Early Adolescence, 1*(2), 185-193.

Lyon, C. 1979. Community services for teen-age mothers. *Human Ecology Forum, 9,* 10-14.

McDonough, S.C. 1984. Effect of assessment results on teen mothers' perspectives of infant development. Paper presented at International Conference on Infant Studies, New York City.

McKenry, P.C., Walters, L.H., & Johnson, C. 1979. Adolescent pregnancy: A review of the literature. *Family Coordinator, 28,* (1), 17-28.

Mednick, B.R., Baker, R.L., & Sutton-Smith, B. (1979). Teenage pregnancy and perinatal mortality. *Journal of Youth and Adolescence, 8*(3), 343-357.

Nakashima, I.I. & Camp, B.W. 1984. Fathers of infants born to adolescent mothers: A study of paternal characteristics. *American Journal of Diseases in the Child, 138,* 452-454.

Nelson, K.G., Key, D., Fletcher, J., Kirkpatrick, E., & Feinstein, R. 1982. The teen-tot clinic: An alternative to traditional care for infants of teenaged mothers. *Journal of Adolescent Health Care, 3*(1), 19-23.

Olds, D.L. 1983. An intervention program for high-risk parents. In R.A. Hackelman (Ed.), *A round table on minimizing high-risk parenting.* Media, Pa.: Harwal Publishing Co., p. 249-268.

Osofsky, H.J., & Osofsky, J.D. 1970. Adolescents as mothers: Results of a program for low-income pregnant teenagers with some emphasis upon infants' development. *American Journal of Orthopsychiatry, 40,* 825-834.

Peabody, E., McKenry, P., & Corders, L. 1981. Subsequent pregnancy among adolescent mothers. *Adolescence, 16*(63), 563-568.

Phipps-Yonas, S. 1980. Teenage pregnancy and motherhood: A review of the literature. *American Journal of Orthopsychiatry, 50*(3), 403-431.

Presser, H.B. 1980. Social consequences of teenage childbearing. In C.S. Chilman (Ed.), *Adolescent pregnancy and childbearing: Findings from research.* U.S. Department of Health and Human Services, Public Health Service, NIH Publication No. 81-2077, p. 249-266.

Ramey, C.T., Collier, A.M., Sparling, J.J., Loda, F.A., Campbell, F.K., Ingram, D.L., & Finkelstein, N.W. 1976. The Carolina Abecedarian Project: A longitudinal and multidisciplinary approach to the prevention of developmental retardation. In T.D. Tjossem (Ed.), *Intervention strategies for high risk infants and young children.* Baltimore: University Park Press, p. 629-668.

Roosa, M., Fitzgerald, H., & Carson, N.A. 1982a. Teenage and older mothers and their infants: A descriptive comparison. *Adolescence, 17*(65), 1-17.

Roosa, M., Fitzgerald, H. & Carson, N.A. 1982b. A comparison of teenage and older mothers: A systems analysis. *Journal of Marriage and the Family, 44,* 367-377.

Sameroff, A.J. 1981. Psychological needs of the mother in early mother-infant interactions. In G.B. Avery (Ed.), *Neonatalogy: Pathophysiology and management of the newborn.* Philadelphia: J.B. Lippincott Co., p. 303-317.

Sameroff, A.J. & Chandler, M.A. 1975. Reproductive risk and the continuum of caretaking casualty. In F.D. Horowitz (Ed.), *Review of Child Development Research,* Vol. 4. Chicago: University of Chicago Press, p. 187-244.

Sandler, H.M. & Vietze, P.M. 1979. Social-psychological characteristics of adolescent mothers and behavioral characteristics of their first-born infants. In K. Scott, T. Field & E. Roberton (Eds.), *Teen-age parents and their offspring.* New York: Grune & Stratton.

Schneider, S. 1982. Helping adolescents deal with pregnancy: A psychiatric approach. *Adolescence, 17*(66), 285-292.

Seitz, V., Apfel, N.H., & Rosenbaum, L.K. 1983. Schoolaged mothers: Infant development and maternal educational outcomes. Paper presented at the Biennial Meeting of the Society for Research in Child Development, Detroit, Michigan.

Smith, E.W. 1975. The role of the grandmother in adolescent pregnancy and parenting. *Journal of School Health, 45*(5), 278-283.

Smith, P.B., Mumford, D.M., & Hamner, E. 1979. Child-rearing attitudes of single teenage mothers. *American Journal of Nursing, 79,* 2115-2116.

Widmayer, S.M., & Field, T.M. 1980. Effects of Brazelton demonstrations on early interactions of preterm infants and their teenage mothers. *Infant Behavior and Development, 3,* 79-89.

Wise, S. & Grossman, F.K. 1980. Adolescent mothers and their infants: Psychological factors in early attachment and interaction. *American Journal of Orthopsychiatry, 50*(3), 454-468.

# Part III

## ISSUES RELATING
## TO STIMULATION AND CONTENT

# Reflections on
# Infant Intervention Programs:
# What Have We Learned?

Alice Sterling Honig, PhD

**ABSTRACT.** Clinical appraisal of model infant intervention projects can inform public policy toward improvement of intervention efforts. Examples of model programs are given; problems that arose are described. Tutorial models focussed on the infant may not impel parents to model the tutorial role. Direct work with parents may not be successful unless tutors are highly skilled. Intensive and extensive therapeutic work with families may be required when an infant is at risk for mental health disturbance. Toddlers in group care behave more aggressively unless prosocial teaching is a prominent curriculum component. Responsive caregiving with infants and strong pride in work enhance staff effectiveness.

Demonstration and research projects over the past decades have implemented a variety of infant intervention models. Many of these federally funded projects had control groups, either randomly assigned or carefully matched with project children on such demographic variables as sex, maternal education and age, ethnicity, birth order and family income. Thus, comparisons could be made between experimental infants and those not in program. One of the successful goals of the earliest projects (such as Keister, 1977 and Caldwell, Wright, Honig, & Tannenbaum, 1970) was to demonstrate the lack of deleterious effects of quality infant group care. Most of the model projects, subsequently, had as their main goal the prevention of cognitive deficits in disadvantaged or handicapped infants. Programs differed on variables such as theoretical rationale, format, evaluation measures, locale (home or educational facility), intensity, presence of parent involvement, and length of intervention (Honig, 1982a).

Alice Sterling Honig is Professor of Child Development at Syracuse University, 201 Slocum Hall, Syracuse, New York 13210.

Most of the infant intervention programs, though not all, showed a significant difference between enriched and control infants on intellective and language scores immediately after programs ended. Yet in many programs, IQ gains washed out over the next few years. Often differences between experimental and control disadvantaged infants were nowhere near as large as the difference between program infants and high-scoring group infants from high-education families. For example, in the Syracuse, N.Y. Family Development Research Program (Honig & Lally, 1982) Center vs. Control IQ scores were 109.97 and 100.77 respectively at 48 months. At that age, infants from high-education contrast groups attained a mean IQ score of 136.05. By six years of age the low income groups no longer differed significantly.

Although IQ gains faded in a few years, satisfactory school achievement and positive societal behaviors (e.g., non-delinquency) have been found to be more characteristic at adolescence for children who had attended the model program as infants or toddlers (Lazar & Darlington, 1982).

## CLINICAL APPRAISAL OF PROGRAMS

In addition to psychometric scores and sociological data, clinical reflections on the historically important demonstration infant enrichment programs of the past decades can be useful in leading to more realistic assessment of the possibilities and limitations of infant intervention. Some families and communities for example, may be too stressed with family violence, drug abuse, and poverty to sustain the loving and learning experiences provided in the best of programs.

More women are entering the labor force and require high quality infant/toddler care. Clinical insights from model projects, in addition to knowledge of relevant child development theory and research findings, can be enlisted in public policy efforts to improve infant enrichment efforts.

## MODEL VARIATIONS: SPECIAL PROBLEMS

Since different kinds of problems arose in different kinds of models, we need to look at the kinds of models that have been tried and evaluated and what some of their special issues were.

*Infant tutoring.* Some early models provided individual tutoring for infants in their own homes (Painter, 1971; Schaefer & Aaronsen, 1977). One of the pitfalls of this model is that the parent may regard the tutor as a convenient free baby sitter. Some parents come to feel that the "expert" knows more about lessons for babies, and that one hour per week with an expert is surely sufficient intellectual activity for a baby. This model has the *potential* for a tutor to serve as a positive role model for parents in daily interactions with infants. In fact, a parent may not perceive this possibility and may not simply "pick up" either the games or the role of tutor.

Some projects provided tutoring for infants in a room in an educational facility. Palmer and Siegel (1977) provided two kinds of interventions for infants in such tutorial sessions. One was *instructional* tutoring on concepts of polar opposites, such as tall-short or wet-dry. The other was a *discovery* experience with toys but without tutoring. A few years after the program ended, preschoolers who had participated in either model were doing equally well on a concept test. Thus, one original expectation of some infant intervention programs (that particular theoretical or curricular models would be more efficacious) was proven untenable in this project.

Other projects, however, did find that one particular curricular model could be more effective than another. Blank and Solomon (1968) carried out Socratic dialogue tutorial sessions with older toddlers in an empty school classroom. Through the use of careful, open ended questions, they taught thinking skills and sequencing of concepts to disadvantaged 36 month olds, (who were deficient in conceptual and language skills) for an hour per day, five days a week for several months. These children made substantial IQ gains in comparison to contrast children who received either no program, a three-day-a-week program, or a daily time for personal attention without the specific reasoning skills curriculum. Thus, particular curricular efforts may indeed make a difference. But this difference may depend on the *training and skills of the tutor* and on the *intensity* with which the tutorial effort is carried out. The tutorial format per se may not guarantee desired cognitive advances.

*Infant group care.* Enriched group care has been the main infant intervention technique in many programs. Some programs have, in addition, offered supports for families, such as infant formula, medical or social work services (Ramey & Campbell, 1981; Caldwell, Wright, Honig & Tannenbaum, 1970). Heber et al. (1972) actively promoted job training for low-income, low IQ mothers as well as initial tutorial infant enrichment at home and then intensive infant enrichment in group care throughout the infancy and preschool years.

A few programs with quality infant group care may be characterized as "omnibus" programs. For example, in Syracuse, New York, The Family Development Research Program (Honig & Lally, 1982) provided infant/toddler day care to enhance self-concept, language, and learning. In addition, a corps of paraprofessional Child Development Trainers brought learning games, positive discipline techniques, nutrition information, and information about community resources and social services to parents during weekly home visits. Book-and-toy lending services and group meetings for parents were also components of the project. This wide array of efforts was designed to prevent intellectual deficit in infants and to help young, low-income, low-education parents become the primary teachers of their own infants and young children. The project goal was to ensure as much as possible the development of positive family social interactions that could, in turn, nurture the program youngsters and provide a firm motivational foundation for their later learning careers in elementary schools.

*Parent based models.* Some programs have opted for teaching parents in groups. Lessons have dealt with how babies grow and learn and what parents can do to impact positively on an infant's development. Badger's work (1977) has taught us that infancy intervention may be more successful with low-education, single, adolescent parents if they are reached in the hospital and enrolled in the program as soon as the baby is born. The perinatal period may be a particularly propitious time for an infant intervention program to enlist young mothers who need support and knowledge and skills so urgently. Young mothers right after birth or even shortly prior to birth may be more open to program ideas and to new ways of thinking about the needs of babies. *Timing* of infancy intervention with the focus on parents may be an important ingredient in success with certain families. Currently, Honig and Pfannenstiel (1983) are testing just this clinical hunch with a program of "Information and Insights about Infants" for low-income first-time fathers whose partners are either in high risk or normal pregnancies.

In other models where families have been the prime target for infancy intervention, *individual home visits* to parents were made. Visitors met parents on territory where the parents were "in charge"—their homes. Parents learned, usually in weekly sessions, how to talk with, read to, and use toys effectively with an infant to promote cognitive and language development (Gordon, Guinagh & Jester, 1977; Lambie, Bond & Weikart, 1974; Levenstein, 1977). In many of these programs, children showed initial IQ gains at end of program and then "washed out" later.

Parent involvement was conceptualized as the key to *sustaining* program gains once a project ended. Yet often, changing a parent's beliefs, understanding, and interactions is a much more complex task than can be accomplished in a brief visit a few times per month.

Some problems and pitfalls were revealed by these program efforts (Honig, 1979).

- —Parents may have *difficulty in seeing themselves as educators* and responsible teaching persons in a child's life.
- —Parents may have *too many personal problems* and too few internal resources for providing the sustained loving and attentive personal interactions required for a child's intellectual thriving.
- —Parents may believe that people always have ulterior, self-serving motives, and so may break appointments, not answer a door bell, and *test the good will of the home visitor* in many ways.
- —Parent involvers may concentrate too much on teaching curriculum for the infant and not enough on helping parents emotionally. Parents need to feel cared about and competent as noticers of newly emerging infant skills, curriculum creators, and effective teacher interactors.
- —Home visitors may not respect alternative life styles, where, for example, infants sleep on blankets on floors rather than in cribs, or toddlers are allowed to stay up to watch late TV shows. *Resentment of parental life style* can hamper the trust-building necessary for change and growth to occur in families.
- —*Parents may change slowly.* Patience and flexibility are absolute necessities for parent program personnel. A program that expects to "home visit" once a month, for a short period of time, and with few specific programmatic goals and procedures, may see very little effect of this intervention (Van Doorninck et al., 1980).
- —*Too many children present* may make the home teaching situation chaotic. Duplicate materials and a partner for home visits may lessen this problem.

—*Differing belief and value systems* between parents and program personnel may increase the likelihood of parental rejection of program ideas. "You spoil a baby if you pick her up", "Children should not talk at meals", "Babies are too young for books", and "You should whip a child to make her behave" are examples that reflect such differences. Research findings can sometimes be used effectively to explain why the program believes and handles certain situations differently from parents.

—*Parents may lack caregiving skills,* so that an infant or toddler is fussy and not amenable to parent lessons. A home visitor can help parents by modelling positive discipline techniques that work and by showing ways to dress and feed that are more comfortable for a child. Such practical assistance may enhance the possibility of more favorable emotional climate for the parent to teach effectively.

—A home visitor may need more sophisticated clinical skills than project training provides in order to carry out home-based work effectively. Fraiberg's (1980) "Kitchen therapy" provided intervention for parents who were inappropriate, neglectful or abusive with infants. A nurturing, perceptive, therapeutic home visitor helped parents get in touch with past griefs and losses. As parents came to trust their relationships with the worker, and began to feel the pain from mistreatment in their own childhood, then they were able to tune into, and interpret correctly, distress signals and needs of their own babies. *Encouragement of insights* as well as educational goals may be necessary.

—Extensive therapeutic family intervention may be necessary to prevent failure to thrive and severe emotional and cognitive deprivation. Thus, some programs provide family services, parent therapy, infant nursery, infant individual therapy, and social service supports such as housing aid and homemaking service (Provence, 1983). The high cost and high practitioner skills required to carry out such programs pose a problem. Whether intervention programs that serve at-risk infants can muster the financial and training resources needed to provide such *extensive* as well as *intensive* therapeutic family services when there is special need is not at all certain under current political and societal priorities.

## THEORETICAL AND RESEARCH BASES
## OF INFANT PROGRAMS

Theoretical ideas and research information form the matrix out of which effective infant programming can develop. Erickson's theory of emotional development (as a succession of resolutions of emotional nuclear conflicts, beginning with the development of basic trust vs. mistrust) and Piaget's equilibration theory are particularly important. Learning is more likely to occur when (1) a child has a rich interactive environment with caring and cared-for persons, and (2) physical materials and experiences are provided in digestible doses so constituted that the equilibration process can successfully occur to promote learning. That is, the infant or toddler struggles and succeeds in making sense of new ideas in the context of what he or she already knows and understands. This active learning process takes place if a caregiver has well-honed "matchmaking" skills (Honig, 1983b). What is new and to be learned by the child cannot be too different, too difficult, too easy, or too novel in comparison with current understandings. Otherwise, the child will not learn—from bewilderment or boredom. Learning encounters need to be finely tuned to a child's current understandings, so that the learning interchanges of adults are sensitive to the infant's response. The caregiver must, as it were, "dance up and down developmental ladders" (Honig, 1982b). If a new idea or skill required seems confusing, a caregiver has to create new ways to make the task a bit simpler. If a toddler finds a task too easy, the caregiver needs to increase difficulty just a bit, so that the joy of the challenge, the child's intrinsic need to master new knowledge and new skills, is enlisted by the adult during teaching interactions.

Certainly, caregivers in infancy intervention projects learned to present educational tasks—to read a book with a baby or to use a toy to encourage language. But Piaget's equilibration theory and Erikson's epigenetic theory require that caregivers be subtly in tune with the intervention *process* in their interactive partnership with infants, not just with curriculum or lesson plans. One can speculate that in some programs, optimal learning transactions that depend on high-level matchmaking skills may not be as prevalent as one would wish. The skills required from the caregiver may not be as available at the salaries paid in the projects. This is a serious and fairly intractable problem in many infant care facilities.

## *EVALUATION OF INFANT INTERVENTION PROJECTS*

A look at the evaluation measures used by infancy intervention projects reveals that intellective and cognitive measures were used overwhelmingly (Honig, 1983a). Some projects did assess infant diets, iron levels, medical status, and classroom social interactions. But infant mental health measures were less likely to be chosen as indices of program success. Given the research findings that positive self-esteem and secure attachment are foundations associated with better problem-solving strategies and ego resilience when toddlers are faced with difficult tasks (Sroufe & Waters, 1977), then it is likely that more assessment emphasis needs to be placed on attachment and socioemotional measures.

Abused toddlers, more and more frequently court-ordered into group care, are more likely to reject friendly adult overtures and act aggressively (Londerville & Main, 1981). *Interactions that result in infant learning may depend more on the quality of the adult-infant relationship and the building of Eriksonian "Basic trust" rather than on fancy toys or elaborate curriculum that a program devises.* Programs need to evaluate the extent of this secure relationship. Some caregivers fall too easily into mistrustful and disapproving patterns well-learned already by toddlers who are accustomed to inappropriate interaction patterns with parents.

Evaluation of programs should be broadened to include attention to questions such as:

— Has the infant/toddler developed a secure, loving relationship with a stable caregiver?
— Do adults present lessons and materials with sensitivity to the particular cognitive developmental level, learning style, tempo and interests of each individual infant or toddler?
— Are lessons embedded in daily routines, which are the meaningful physical and psychological landmarks of an infant's daily experiences?
— Are lessons always separate (i.e., encapsulated language or math sessions) or are content and concepts generalized to mundane yet personal, intimate daily activities such as diapering and feeding?
— Are prosocial skills part of the infant group care curriculum? Finkelstein (1982) has reported higher aggression scores for preschoolers after early day care.

—Do the caregivers respond to infant initiatives and recognize the teachable moment when a learning activity may be underway that an adult can profitably build upon?

An example of subtle problems in implementing program goals may illuminate the need for *process* as well as outcome measures:

A mother, who had learned in a parent-focused project that book reading was very important with toddlers, was videotaped while reading with her toddler. They sat close together on a couch and mother had one arm around Timmy. "Look at the orange", she urged. The toddler was silent. "See the orange. Say orange", she continued vigorously. The orange was the top picture of the right-hand page of an opened picture book on their laps. Timmy's eyes were riveted to a horse with a flowing mane on the left-hand page, "Come on. Say orange!" repeatedly urged the mother in a firm, pleasant tone. Finally, while still looking at the horse with the flowing mane, Timmy said mechanically "Orange." Instead of then talking about oranges, or asking the child to tell her about the picture or about a real orange in his experience, the mother immediately moved her eyes and her teaching efforts to the lemon pictured just underneath the orange. "O.K. Honey. Here's a lemon. Say lemon", she urged cheerfully. Timmy's eyes were still enjoying the flowing mane and tail of the horse on the opposite page. The noticing skills of the teaching person and the process of the teaching interaction may be far more important for cognitive enhancement of infants and toddlers than a particular curricular procedure. In some parent-focussed programs, adult cognitive ability to devise and revise teaching strategies contingent on an infant's responses may be as problematic as their ability to nurture emotionally. These issues need to be faced in carrying out and evaluating program.

## THE SOCIAL PSYCHOLOGY OF INTERVENTION: AN IMPORTANT FACTOR

Child caregiving is a profession that requires dedication, emotional sensitivity to children, intellectually accurate decoding of child communications, appropriate responsivity, and high energy.

Even in high-quality infant intervention projects, caregivers were often poorly paid. Those who worked with families often found the stress debilitating.

In addition, some caregivers, due to job turnover and program needs, were not as well trained as others. Caregivers with less training are not as responsive to cues or bids from children. Honig and Wittmer (1982; in press), in a study of metropolitan day care teachers and toddlers, report that 20-30% of toddler bids (for attention, help, information, etc.) were not responded to by the teacher. Most toddlers abandoned their interactive bid when ignored. Some persisted. One ingenious toddler asked, "Where dis go?" as he held up a puzzle piece to the teacher. After being ignored several times in this bid, the toddler held the puzzle piece over a basin and asked "Go in dere?" This action brought a response! "No, put it in your puzzle", the teacher stated firmly.

Ongoing training for infant/toddler teachers is an absolute necessity for morale building and for professional growth. Even caregivers who had received intensive preservice training in the Syracuse project required "renewal". There is a drift downward, a kind of "burn out", that can occur in daily work with very young children who need constant care and attention. Thus, infant/toddler intervention programs need to build in not only coffee breaks and floating "helper" staff for group care, but also training time and money. This may require political lobbying and public pressure for civic funds to support training.

Caregivers need to hear new ideas that work with babies, see new books and new films about infant development. They need time to dialogue about infant problems, time to plan and carry out toy making, time to invent new ways to arrange classroom environments to encourage active learning. They need to learn what infant signals might mean, what techniques will enhance early pleasureful language communications, how to prolong attention and persistence in learning games; how to respond to infant initiatives so that babies feel good about their own persons and can learn well. Easy to read materials for infant/toddler training abound (Honig, 1981, 1983b; 1984; Honig & Lally 1981; Willis & Ricciuti, 1975).

When caregivers feel the importance of their work, they become more motivated. They feel part of an important societal effort, for example, to help prevent cognitive deficit in disadvantaged infants, or to add to the peace of mind of a single working parent who is try-ing to make a living for her family. Helping staff (1) feel connected with an important societal job, (2) feel trained to make such contributions, and (3) feel their contributions are intangible yet priceless ingredients that can improve the quality of infant care programs.

## REFERENCES

Badger, E.D. (1977). *Postnatal classes for high risk mother-infant pairs.* Cincinnati: University of Cincinnati College of Medicine.

Blank, M. & Solomon, F. (1968). A tutorial language program to develop abstract thinking in socially disadvantaged preschool children. *Child Development, 39,* 279-389.

Caldwell, B.M., Wright, C.M., Honig, A.S., Tannenbaum, J. (1970). Infant day care and attachment. *American Journal of Orthopsychiatry, 40,* 397-412.

Finkelstein, N. (1982). Aggression: Is it stimulated by day care? *Young Children, 37,* 3-13.

Fraiberg, S. (1980). *Clinical studies of infant mental health: The first year of life.* New York: Basic Books.

Gordon I., Guinagh, B., & Jester, R. (1977). The Florida parent education infant toddler programs. In M.C. Day & R.K. Parker (Eds.), *The preschool in action* (2nd ed.). Boston: Allyn & Bacon.

Heber, R., Garber, H., Harrington, S. & Hoffman, C. (1972). *Rehabilitation of families at risk for mental retardation:* A progress report. Madison: University of Wisconsin.

Honig, A.S. (1979). *Parent involvement in early childhood education* (Rev. ed.). Washington, D.C.: National Association for the Education of Young Children.

Honig, A.S. (1981). What are the needs of infants? *Young Children, 37,* 3-10.

Honig, A.S. (1982a). Intervention strategies to optimize infant development. In E. Aronowitz (Ed.), *Prevention strategies for mental health.* New York: Neale Watson Academic Publishers.

Honig, A.S. (1982b). *Playtime learning games for young children.* Syracuse, New York: Syracuse University Press.

Honig, A.S. (1983a). Evaluation of infant/toddler intervention programs. In B. Spodek (Ed.), *Studies in education evaluation.* London: Pergamon Press.

Honig, A.S. (1983b). Meeting the needs of infants. *Dimensions, 11*(2), 4-7.

Honig, A.S. (1984). Quality training for infant caregivers, *Child Care Quarterly, 12*(2), 121-135.

Honig, A.S. & Lally, J.R. (1981). *Infant caregiving: A design for training.* Syracuse, New York: Syracuse University Press.

Honig, A.S. & Lally, J.R. (1982). The Family Development Research Program: Retrospective review. *Early Child Development and Care, 10,* 42-62.

Honig, A.S. & Pfannenstiel, A. (1983). *Effects of a prenatal "Infancy Information/Support Curriculum" on fathers' post-natal attitudes, knowledge, self-image as a father, and interaction with their infants following either a high or low risk pregnancy.* Syracuse University Senate Research Committee Grant. Syracuse University, Syracuse, New York.

Honig, A.S. & Wittmer, D.S. (1982). Teachers and low-income toddlers in metropolitan day care. *Early Child Development and Care, 10,* 95-112.

Honig, A.S. & Wittmer, D.S. (in press). Toddler bids and teacher responses. *Child Care Quarterly.*

Keister, M. (1977). *"The good life" for infants and toddlers: Group care of infants (2nd ed.).* Washington, D.C.: National Association for the Education of Young Children.

Lambie, D., Bond, J.F. & Weikart, D. (1974). *Home teaching with mothers and infants.* Ypsilanti, Michigan: High/Scope Educational Research Foundation.

Lazar, I. & Darlington, R. (1982). Lasting effects of early education: A report from the consortium for longitudinal studies. *Monographs of the Society for Research in Child Development, 45* (Nos. 2 & 3), Serial No. 195.

Levenstein, P. (1977). The mother-child home program. In M.C. Day & R.D. Parker (Eds.), *The preschool in action: Exploring early childhood programs.* Boston: Allyn & Bacon.

Londerville, S. & Main, M. (1981). Security of attachment, compliance, and maternal training methods in the second year of life. *Developmental Psychology, 17,* 289-299.

Painter, G. (1971). *Teach your baby.* New York: Simon & Schuster.

Palmer, F. & Siegel, R. (1977). Minimal intervention at ages two and three and subsequent intellective changes. In M. Day & R.D. Parker (Eds.), *The preschool in action* (2nd ed.). Boston: Allyn & Bacon.

Provence, S. (Ed.). (1983). *Infants and parents: Clinical case reports.* New York: International Universities Press.

Ramey, C. & Campbell, F.A. (1981). Educational intervention for children at risk for mild retardation: A longitudinal analysis. In P. Mittler (Ed.), *Frontiers of knowledge in mental retardation.* Baltimore: University Park Press.

Schaefer, E. & Aaronson, M. (1977). Infant education research project: Implementation and implications of a home tutoring program. In M. Day & R.D. Parker (Eds.), *The preschool in action.* Boston: Allyn & Bacon.

Sroufe, L.A. & Waters, E. (1977). Attachment as an organizational construct. *Child Development, 48,* 1194-1199.

Van Doorninck, W.J., Dawson, P., Butterfield, P. & Alexander, M.I. (1980). *Parent-infant support through lay health visitors.* Final Report. Denver: Parent Infant Programs.

Willis, A. & Ricciuti, H. (1975). *A good beginning for babies: Guidelines for group care.* Washington, D.C.: National Association for the Education of Young Children.

# Relationship of Infant Psychobiological Development to Infant Intervention Programs

Judith M. Gardner, PhD
Bernard Z. Karmel, PhD
John M. Dowd, PhD

**ABSTRACT.** The present paper offers some cautions concerning potential risks involved in prescribing intervention when it is not necessary and potential problems with matching the nature of intervention to the characteristics and developmental level of individual infants. It is our position that intervention should only be attempted when the infant is at risk for poor outcome because early stimulation as a means to enhance development may not always be beneficial for adaptive functioning at later ages. We describe two fundamental psychobiological aspects of behavior during early infancy, state organization and attention to stimulation, and stress the importance of understanding such functioning with respect to preterm and CNS damaged infants as well as healthy infants.

## I. PROBLEMS AND ISSUES

In general, healthy fullterm infants are born with most of their physiological systems coordinated and well-adapted to the immediate environment they are likely to face after birth. This structural and functional organization of the infant is evident in the fundamental processes of state modulation and attention to stimulation that are necessary antecedent conditions to learning and cognitive growth. In the present paper, we will briefly describe these processes during the first few months of life. In so doing, we will em-

Judith M. Gardner and John M. Dowd are Lecturers and Bernard Z. Karmel is Associate Professor in the Departments of Pediatrics and Psychiatry, Mt. Sinai Medical Center, New York, New York.

Requests for reprints should be sent to Judith M. Gardner, Department of Pediatrics, Annenberg 17-80, Mt. Sinai Medical Center, 1 Gustave Levy Place, New York, New York 10029.

*93*

phasize the differences in functioning between young and older infants; and how infants born at risk for poor developmental outcome, especially very low birthweight (VLBW) infants, might deviate from the basic pattern. We will try to show the importance of understanding infant functioning in the context of early stimulation programs.

Our position is that early intervention can be either beneficial or harmful depending on the appropriateness of the program to the characteristics of the baby, the environment, and the transactions between them. Traditionally, infant intervention programs have adopted the tacit position that more stimulation is better. We propose that this is not always the case; that there is an optimal level or amount of stimulation for individual babies, which is jointly determined by internal and external sources of stimulation. Increasing environmental stimulation is not necessarily beneficial and, under certain circumstances, may even be detrimental. Thus, nonspecific early infant stimulation programs are potentially harmful if the intensity and type of stimulation are not tailored to the needs of individual infants.

There is currently a popular trend toward "education" in early infancy even when the infant has no identifiable biological or environmental reason for being at risk for normal development. The rationale for this advocacy is that, even if a particular infant is normal and healthy and is being cared for in a responsive environment and so not in need of intervention, the program can only help. In our view, this type of thinking is naive and overlooks some potential risks. For those infants who are normal and healthy, intervention will be superfluous at best. Despite the heralded claims of some, there are no programs established to date that have been proven capable beyond any doubt of making normal healthy babies into "super babies". Healthy normal babies cared for in a supportive responsive environment develop quite well without intervention. To recommend a program for such an infant is not logical even if such programs have proved helpful in cases where central nervous system (CNS) damage is documented or has been suspected (e.g., chronic or acute CNS insults such as intrauterine hypoxia or birth asphyxia leading to brain hemorrhage). In fact, the imposition of "intervention" by well-meaning health practitioners and educators when there are no indications of dysfunction or pathology may have questionable consequences by creating the false perception in the parents that what they are doing is inadequate or that their normal baby could become a "super baby" with the program but certainly could not without the program. Parents not enrolled in such programs for whatever reasons may lower their expectations for their infant and create a self-fulfilling prophecy of failure. A related problem is that of how to intervene for the baby who is known to have suffered CNS insult leading to chronic impairment. The common strategy has been to heroically attempt to keep the baby's progress from falling behind expectations based on population norms. This can also have questionable consequences for all involved by raising expectations too high, producing a situation where failure may be the outcome.

Although there has been a recent impetus in the field of early education toward early stimulation programs, their effectiveness is extremely difficult to evaluate. Such programs are typically evaluated solely in terms of whether or not they are effective in enhancing the development of the participant infants, with the sensitive question of whether infant stimulation programs can possibly be harmful never being addressed. Frequently, the lack of adverse outcome in many high risk infants who were suspected of having significant CNS insult and subsequently received intervention is cited as "proof" that early intervention is beneficial. Unfortunately, such encouraging results do not constitute proof of effectiveness. What is being overlooked is the plasticity of the developing CNS and the amount of uncertainty of most diagnoses (except for extremely damaged babies) due to insufficient information to confirm the exact character and degree of CNS insult that may have occurred. Thus, good outcome could have occurred anyway with normal experience in a healthy environment and without "infant stimulation". Without appropriate baseline data with which to make comparisons, it is impossible to determine the true efficacy of any program. This is not to say that programs never should be recommended for infants whose exact status is in doubt. Rather, we wish to call into question indiscriminate recommendations for early stimulation, and to urge caution and careful consideration.

## II. PSYCHOBIOLOGICAL FUNCTIONING IN HIGH RISK NEONATES: ISSUES IN PREDICTING OUTCOME

If intervention is not to be universally recommended, then how shall we decide when and how to intervene? To answer this question it is essential to first consider some of the issues involved when insult is evident during the neonatal period and how such insult might alter the normal course of development. Over the past two decades medical progress in prenatal, perinatal, and postnatal care has dramatically improved the survival rate of immature and sick infants. These advances have changed the nature of the population of at risk infants as well as the severity and types of development problems incurred. In VLBW infants, the incidence of major neurological defects appears to be decreasing (Davies & Tizard, 1975), while the incidence of more subtle cognitive and perceptual dysfunctions appears to have increased (Caputo, Goldstein, & Taub, 1981; Grellong, Vaughan, Rotkin, Daum, Kurtzberg, & Lipper, 1981; Kitchen, Ryan, Richards, McDougall, Billson, Keir, & Naylor, 1980; see also Rie & Rie, 1980). Discovering the specific reasons for these more subtle effects requires not only understanding CNS function and organization, but how such atypical early experiences as immaturity and illness are expressed in altered development of brain structure and activity as well as behavioral performance. Such knowledge should be a fundamental precursor to any infant stimulation program designed to ameliorate the effects of early insults.

Furthermore, preterms, healthy or otherwise, are not just immature fullterm infants. They are not born with their physiological systems coordinated and well-adapted for extrauterine life as are healthy fullterm babies. Most also have been significantly stressed. The nature of prematurity and early illness, as well as the iatrogenic effects of medical procedures and environmental conditions on a Neonatal Intensive Care Unit, are such that once stressful conditions occur they alter the course and duration of subsequent developmental sequences. Atypical early experiences do not simply interfere with the organization of an already mature system. Instead, because of the plasticity of the developing nervous system and the dynamic transactional nature of developmental processes, early experiences can rearrange functional connection in the brain which is itself changing. The reorganization and redirection of all aspects of development can be the resultant consequence.

Preterm and sick neonates are a very heterogeneous population of infants. In addition, knowledge is limited concerning how specific medical problems, interacting with different medical treatments and/or environmental conditions, relate to subsequent outcome. For that matter, what appear to be major deviations in structural and functional organization may alter the course of development but not necessarily prevent normality from eventually occurring. Many examples exist in which seemingly devastating insults in infancy, such as hydrocephalus, are associated with relatively good outcome (Giuffre, Palma, & Fontana, 1979; Griffith & Davidson, 1966; McFie, 1961; Piercy, 1964).

There is support for transactional processes (Sameroff & Chandler, 1975) accounting for why some risk infants have later dysfunction while others do not. For example, evidence for the ameliorating effect of social interactions comes from an ongoing longitudinal study by Parmelee and co-workers (Parmelee, Beckwith, Cohen, & Sigman, 1983). They show that outcome is only indirectly related to pre and postnatal complications or medical problems during infancy. It is also mediated by the quality of mother-infant interaction, which in turn is affected by the status of the infant at birth. Thus, conditions such as prematurity and early illness which are markedly deviant with respect to both experiential and biological factors may produce only subtle or small deviations from normal functioning at older ages.

Unfortunately, the converse may also be true in that factors which appear to have only minor or transient effects at the time they occur very early in life may be amplified to become major difficulties later on (Hebb, 1942; Parmelee, 1975; Schneider, 1979; Thoman, 1981). For example, the variability of bradycardia, respiration, and apnea in presumably healthy babies may be manifestations of immaturity or disorganization in the brainstem or associated regions, the result of which could be sudden infant death syndrome, seizures, or attention disorders at older ages.

Given these alternative possibilities, a host of developmental uncertainties arise. These uncertainties must be considered in decisions regarding the need for early intervention or stimulation programs, their possible effects on different babies, and the types of therapies that should be undertaken. This is especially true because, even though there is some available research with babies, the effects of various types of early stimulation on individual infants have not been well delineated. The animal literature, however, provides relevant information from a variety of studies.

## III. EARLY STIMULATION EFFECTS ON CNS DEVELOPMENT: ANIMAL STUDIES

There are numerous animal studies related to the issues of early stimulation and the interaction of biological and environmental factors on development. We will briefly describe representative studies that emphasize particularly important aspects of the effects of early stimulation on both general and specific areas of nervous system development that sometimes are overlooked in a simplistic approach to early intervention.

First, too much or too little enhancement of general nervous system development appears, for the most part, to be detrimental. This is an important point because one goal of stimulation programs is to increase the amount of information acquired by the infant through enhancement or acceleration of CNS development. For example, a series of studies has been reported, using rat pups, on the effects of too little or too much thyroxin, the hormone secreted by the thyroid gland that plays an integral role in the rate of CNS maturation and behavioral development (Davenport & Gonzalez, 1973; Eayres, 1971; Shapiro, 1968; Shapiro & Norman, 1967). With hypothyroidism, or too little thyroxin, development is retarded and there are intellectual deficits. If excess thyroxin is given to infant rats, CNS development initially appears to be enhanced, as judged by acceleration of neuroanatomical and neurochemical systems, as well as by acceleration of behavioral development such as eye opening, reflexes, and other locomotor responses. However, when these advanced rat pups become older, they show impairment of learning capacity in contrast to normal pups. Thus, a seemingly beneficial effect in the short term appears to have deleterious consequences in the long term, possibly due to alteration of the phasing of CNS maturational processes.

Second, enhancement of specific aspects of CNS functioning, such as in the sensory systems, also appears to be detrimental. Sensory system development is a finely tuned process which is well adapted for functioning in the normal case. It appears to be highly dependent on the different senses receiving appropriate input at appropriate levels of maturity. For example, recent work with rat pups shows that too early eye opening can produce disruptions in the development of sensory systems and their hierarchical relationships (Kenny & Turkewitz, 1983). Before the normal time of eye opening, rat pups find their home nest through olfactory cues. After their eyes open they use vision and also show decreased orientation to the nest. If their eyes surgically are opened earlier than normal, the pups show an initial facilitation of the visual system. However, when visual cues are then not available, there are deficits in their ability to use olfactory cues and the normal decline in response to the nest does not occur as it does at the time of the normal shift from olfaction to vision. Moreover, at older ages, the rats show impaired visual learning. Again, a procedure that initially appears to have facilitating effects subsequently produces deficits. There are analogous findings in humans. Preterm infants are exposed to visual stimulation at earlier ages than fullterms who are without such stimulation until birth. It was originally believed that such early stimulation should enhance visual system development. However, this does not occur. Preterms tend to have more variable and disorganized visual responses rather than more mature ones (Parmelee, 1975). Thus, as with global acceleration of CNS development through biochemical manipulations, additional stimulation of a specific area such as the visual system through environmental manipulations, may be disruptive or deleterious to achieving normal adaptive functioning at maturity.

## IV. ATTENTION:
## AN IMPORTANT PSYCHOBIOLOGICAL EFFECT
## ON EARLY FUNCTION

A basic understanding of the characteristics of the infant thus is primary in order to decide which babies might benefit from intervention, what types of intervention might be appropriate, and what predictions might be made about possible effects and outcomes. In this respect, an understanding of young infants' attentional behavior and the factors contributing to it is essential.

Newborn infants are capable of responding to input from a variety of sensory modalities. They respond differentially to visual patterns such as checkerboards containing different sizes and numbers of checks, to auditory stimuli containing different phonemes such as "ba" and "pa", to different tastes such as sweet or bitter, and so on. Thus, in recent years, the neonate has been portrayed as the "competent" infant. However, the bases for such discriminations appear to change with development. The same responses have different meaning and significance when made by very young as opposed to older infants; and similarities to older infants' behavior are often more apparent than real. Care must therefore be taken not to assume that just because young babies can discriminate along many interesting environmental dimensions of stimulation, they are necessarily doing so on the same basis as older infants or children.

During the neonatal period, infant attention appears to be more a function of the overall amount of stimulation, whether internal or external in origin, than to any specific properties or features of the stimuli. Furthermore, and most importantly, this total amount of stimulation has been shown to be jointly determined by physical properties of the stimulus and by organismic variables, the latter including the nature and state of the receptors and the general arousal level of the infant (see Gardner & Karmel, 1983; Schneirla, 1965; Turkewitz, Gardner, & Lewkowicz, 1984; Turkewitz, Lewkowicz, & Gardner, 1983 for further exposition of the theoretical perspective and studies germane to this point).

Studies of visual attention provide much of the supporting evidence for this view. Much of this research uses the visual preference technique in which two pictures or objects are shown simultaneously to the baby, while measuring how long the baby looks at each. Looking preferences as measures of early attentional mechanisms have typically been discussed in relation to univariate quantitative dimensions of stimulation such as brightness, number of angles, size and number of elements, contour density, and spatial and temporal frequency (Fantz & Fagan, 1975). However, variations along any single dimension do not totally account for the looking preferences of very young infants. Most likely the dimensions interact, so that looking is determined by some combined or multivariate effect. For example, in infants younger than two months of age, contour density preferences can be altered by changing the brightness of the stimulus, which is not the case in older infants (McCarvill & Karmel, 1976). In the same manner, when presented with patterned stimuli such as bulls-eyes or stripes, infants who are less than ten weeks of age exhibit visual preferences based upon size (Maisel & Karmel, 1978; Ruff & Turkewitz, 1975) and brightness (Ruff & Turkewitz, 1979), whereas older infants exhibit preferences that can be based on pattern configuration. Furthermore, exposure to quantitative variations in stimulation either from other modalities or from differences in arousal levels also exert systematic effects on neonates' visual preferences. For instance, when white noise is presented concurrently with visual stimuli, neonates prefer fewer cubes than when no noise is presented (Lawson & Turkewitz, 1980); and neonates previously exposed to white noise prefer lights of a lower luminance level than babies not exposed to noise (Lewkowicz & Turkewitz, 1981). Similarly, neonates initially exposed to white noise pulsing at faster temporal frequencies subsequently prefer looking at lights flashing at slower frequencies than do babies either initially exposed to noise pulsing at slower frequencies or not exposed to noise (Gardner, Lewkowicz, & Rose, 1983). Finally, changes in level of arousal influence visual attention in much the same way as modification of external sources of stimulation. That is, neonates' contour and temporal frequency preferences change as a function of their internal state such that when more aroused, neonates prefer looking at less stimulating events and, when less aroused, they prefer looking at more stimulating events (Gardner & Karmel, 1983; Gardner & Turkewitz, 1982).

## V. AROUSAL AND ITS RELATIONSHIP TO ATTENTION: IMPORTANT PSYCHOBIOLOGICAL EFFECTS ON EARLY FUNCTION

Infants cannot gain information, learn about the world, or interact socially, unless they first attend to relevant features or their environment. In so doing, they are active participants and not just passive recipients of input. Unfortunately, most research on infant attention including our earlier work (cf. Karmel & Maisel, 1975) has emphasized characteristics of the stimulus, and generally has considered the baby merely a passive entity that is affected by stimulation. As long as the baby is awake and attending, the baby's internal state or arousal level is not considered to be important. However, if the baby is an active participant in the determination of his or her looking preferences, it seems reasonable to assume that internal changes or differences within the baby are also likely to affect responding to visual stimuli.

Given that there is some preferred level of stimulation that maximizes orienting toward a particular stimulus, and that this level is dependent on the contribution of both external and internal sources of stimulation, any change in the overall amount of stimulation (from whatever source) should alter what the baby attends to. Thus, a stimulus that is preferred when the baby is in a quiet attending state may not be preferred when the baby is at a different arousal level. Moreover, infants normally behave in such a way as to maintain their optimal level of arousal. That is, because biological systems tend to be homeostatic, the combined effects of external and internal factors must reach some maximal or optimal limit (Karmel & Maisel, 1975), thereby producing a directional relationship. In other words, when a baby is more aroused, and has higher levels of internal activity, he or she should orient toward a less intense stimulus, and when a baby is less aroused and has lower levels of internal activity, he or she should orient toward a more intense stimulus (see Field, 1981; Gardner & Karmel, 1983).

The extremes of this inverse relationship are fairly well known, as when a sleeping baby responds only to fairly intense stimulation, or a highly aroused baby shuts down or turns away from almost all incoming stimuli. If our interest is in understanding and promoting active, awake involvement of the baby with the environment, it is even more important to study this relationship within a more restricted range of arousal levels when the baby is awake. Although investigators of infant behavior have repeatedly recognized the importance of internal state and arousal level in determining the amount and kind of responding to stimulation (Als, Lester, & Brazelton, 1979; Parmelee, 1975; Prechtl, 1974; Thoman, 1981), there is little systematic knowledge of how normal fluctuations in internal state affect reactions to external stimulation. However, this can readily be studied through manipulation of the baby's feeding and swaddling conditions. Since both feeding (Clifton, 1978; Korner, 1972) and swaddling (Lipton, Steinschneider, & Richmond, 1965) have been shown to reduce internal levels of activity, the arousal changes produced by these normally occurring events can be used to study the effects of arousal on specific behaviors such as looking preferences.

We operationalized and evaluated this hypothesis in a series of studies with preterm and fullterm neonates and found systematic relationships between arousal level and visual preferences. The preterm infants we studied were tested close to the time they should have been born. Whey they were less aroused (after feeding and while swaddled), they preferred stimuli having more cubes or a faster temporal frequency than when they were more aroused (before feeding and while unswaddled) (Gardner & Turkewitz, 1982). Fullterm neonates demonstrated a similar inverse relationship between arousal level and temporal frequency (Gardner & Karmel, 1984). These infants preferred faster frequencies when they were less aroused and slower frequencies when they were more aroused.

We could postulate that CNS damage is likely to fundamentally alter the normal internal state organization of the baby. Given that this occurs, what would be "stimulating" to the normal infant, would not necessarily be "stimulating" to the same degree to the dysfunctional or CNS-damaged infant due to deficits in internal state-modulating capacities.

## VI. ATTENTION AND AROUSAL SYSTEMS IN PRETERM INFANTS

In the preterm infant, the immaturity of the nervous system and differing degrees of adaptive readiness of various subsystems appear to be manifested biologically in structural problems such as intraventricular bleeding, and functionally in a lack of state organization. The items on neuro-behavioral assessments tend to bear out these differences. Most frequently, items that differentiate the preterm from the fullterm infant are those that deal with interactive processes and state organization (although motoric processes can also be important depending on the nature of the insult) (Brazelton, Als, Tronick, & Lester, 1979; Kurtzberg, Daum, Grellong, Albin, & Rotkin, 1979). These types of internal mechanisms relating state organization to behavioral and CNS integration have been proposed to explain differences in interactions with objects and people at later ages (Field, 1979).

Modulation of state has been proposed by a number of investigators to explain early functioning. In this manner, not only would too much or too little arousal affect performance on such tasks as orienting and attending, but variations in responding to the same external stimulus would be determined, in part, by the infant's capacity to modulate arousal through these orienting and attending behaviors. For example, Sroufe (1979) proposed a "tension release" model in which affective behaviors such as gaze aversion and smiling help the infant to modulate arousal. Field (1981) indicated the need to include organismic variables such as state and developmental change in this type of model. She has extended and combined Sroufe's "tension release" model with Sokolov's (1963) model of orienting and defensive responses to show that preterm infants exhibit a limited range of stimulation to which they will respond optimally (Field, 1981). Preterms tend to show a higher threshold for response to low-intensity stimuli and a lower threshold or disorganized responding to higher intensity stimuli. This state of affairs can produce a situation documented by Field (1979) in which the behavior of mothers of preterms can, in fact, be counterproductive. She found that mothers tend to overstimulate their nonresponsive infants, who then are more likely to become overaroused. Overaroused infants avert their gaze, thereby eliciting greater efforts from their mothers to attract their attention. The end result of such a vicious cycle, if uninterrupted, can only be a feeling on the part of the mother that everything she does is wrong or that the baby does not like her.

Our work with attention and arousal systems in preterms and fullterms, although not specifically designed to evaluate differences between babies, did suggest some qualitative differences that would be important to know in specific detail with respect to intervention or stimulation. For instance, preterms tended to show more variable behavior. The variability between babies was much greater. They were much more difficult to test than fullterms. In general, testing took longer because they did not remain in a quiet, alert state as well, and more interruptions were required to bring them to an appropriate state for testing. Finally, preterm infants displayed more "shut down" behavior to stimulus onset than did fullterms. In fact, in fullterms, with comparable stimuli, this behavior is rarely observed. Most fullterms have a behavior known as "locking on". They fixate a visual stimulus and continue to look at the stimulus for a long time, sometimes never shifting their gaze to the other stimulus which has been simultaneously presented. Preterms typically did not show this "locking on" behavior, and were much more likely to flit back and forth between stimuli, giving them an increased number of shorter looks. At older ages, this type of behavior would indicate maturity of the nervous system because infants who do not "lock on" are able to release their gaze when they so desire, especially if they get bored looking at the same stimulus. In preterms, however, the absence of "locking on" is more likely to indicate immaturity and lack of integrity of the nervous system.

In general, preterms did show the effects of feeding and swaddling on looking preferences. But, unlike the fullterms, there were some infants who did not. Unfortunately, the sample size was not large enough to try to precisely identify which pre or postnatal factors might have been related to this. However, a correlation between total number of obstetric and postnatal problems and shifts in looking preferences with shifts in arousal level was observed. The more problems a baby had, the less likely was the feeding and swaddling condition to affect looking preferences.

We know that not all preterms have problems, and this is true even for the very small ones. The difficult task remains identifying those babies who are more likely to have future problems and differentiating them from those who are not. Although most preterms have problems with state modulating capacities, those who do not shift their behavior, even with the aid of externally imposed conditions such as feeding and swaddling, may be at much greater risk. Furthermore, these infants are the very ones that are likely to be most vulnerable to being overstimulated or overwhelmed by poorly designed programs that simply seek to provide maximal levels of stimulation as "enrichment". Therefore, it seems essential not only to identify such babies by evaluating their response characteristics in the context of changing arousal level, but also to design individual programs appropriate for them.

## VII. CONCLUSION

We hope that the foregoing discussion sufficiently emphasizes the importance of the fundamental processes of state modulation and attention to stimulation during early infancy as they relate to the issue of infant stimulation and intervention. For programs to be beneficial and avoid potentially harmful complications, it is important to understand the nature of these processes in early infancy; how they change with development; and how, through the process of transactions between the infant and the environment, perinatal insults to the CNS can alter the normal course of development. An understanding of these factors is, we feel, a basic prerequisite to the design of any sound intervention program.

We purposefully have not addressed the many issues concerning environmentally deficient homes, although we certainly appreciate their significance. Instead, we have focussed our discussion on risk factors associated with prematurity and early illness. We take a stand against the position that normal healthy infants cared for in supportive responsive environments would necessarily benefit from early stimulation programs. A key principle that we have tried to stress is that young infants respond to the total amount of stimulation present rather than to qualitative dimensions or specific features of external stimuli; and, furthermore, that this total amount of stimulation is jointly determined by both external and internal sources. Thus, the optimal level of stimulation will be different for different infants.

It follows from these arguments that more stimulation is not necessarily better and can, in fact, be detrimental. The animal literature provides strong support for this position, indicating that both the amount of stimulation and the developmental sequencing of modalities of stimulation have important influences on the early course of development. Studies with human infants also support this position, although the evidence is less extensive. For those infants who appear to require intervention, care must be taken that the program is appropriate to their developmental stage, state modulating characteristics, and capabilities. Moreover, frequent reassessments and adjustments should be made as the infant progresses. Finally, it should be emphasized, preterm and very sick infants represent a particularly sensitive population. Because these infants tend to have more disorganized and less coherent nervous systems, special care must be taken in considering what infant stimulation is mandated.

## REFERENCES

Als, H., Lester, B.M., & Brazelton, T.B. (1979). Dynamics of the behavioral organization of the premature infant: A theoretical perspective. In T. Field, A. Sostek, S. Goldberg, & H.H. Shuman (Eds.), *Infants born at risk: Behavior and development.* New York: Spectrum.

Brazelton, T.B., Als, H., Tonick, E., & Lester, B.M. (1979). Specific neonatal measures: The Brazelton Neonatal Behavior Assessment Scale. In J. Osofsky (Ed.), *Handbook of infant development.* New York: Wiley.

Caputo, D.V., Goldstein, K.M., & Taub, H.B. (1981). The development of prematurely born children through middle childhood. In S. Friedman & M. Sigman (Eds.), *Preterm birth and psychological development.* New York: Academic Press.

Clifton, R. (1978). The relation of infant cardiac responding to behavioral state and motor activity. In W.A. Collins (Ed.), *Minnesota Symposia on Child Psychology* (Vol. 11). Hillsdale, N.J.: Lawrence Erlbaum.

Davenport, J.W., & Gonzalez, L.M. (1973). Neonatal thyroxine stimulation in rats: Accelerated behavioral maturation and subsequent learning deficit. *Journal of Comparative and Physiological Psychology, 85,* 397-408.

Davies, P.A., & Tizard, J.P.M. (1975). Very low birthweight and subsequent neurological defect (with special reference to spastic diplegia). *Developmental Medicine and Child Neurology, 17,* 3-17.

Eayres, J.T. (1971). Thyroid and developing brain: Anatomical and behavioral deficits. In M. Hamburgh & E.J.W. Barrington (Eds.), *Hormones in development.* New York: Appleton-Century-Crofts.

Fantz, R.L., & Fagan, J.F. (1975). Visual attention to size and number of pattern details by term and preterm infants during the first six months. *Child Development, 46,* 3-18.

Field, T. (1979). Interaction patterns of high-risk and normal infants. In T. Field, A. Sostek, S. Goldberg, & H.H. Shuman (Eds.), *Infants born at risk: Behavior and development.* New York: Sprectrum.

Field, T. (1981). Infant arousal, attention, and affect during early interactions. In L. Lipsitt & C. Rovee-Collier (Eds.), *Advances in infancy research* (Vol. 1). Norwood, N.J.: Ablex.

Gardner, J.M., & Karmel, B.Z. (1983). Attention and arousal in preterm and fullterm neonates. In T. Field & A. Sostek (Eds.), *Infants born at risk: Physiological, perceptual, and cognitive processes.* New York: Grune & Stratton.

Gardner, J.M., & Karmel, B.Z. (1984). Arousal effects on visual preferences in neonates. *Developmental Psychology, 20,* 374-377.

Gardner, J.M., Lewkowicz, D.J., & Rose, S.A. (1983, April). Effects of prestimulation on visual preferences in neonates. Paper presented at the biennial meeting of the Society for Research in Child Development, Detroit.

Gardner, J.M., & Turkewitz, G. (1982). The effect of arousal level on visual preferences in preterm infants. *Infant Behavior and Development, 5,* 369-385.

Giuffre, R., Palma, L., & Fontana, M. (1979). Extracranial CSF shunting for infantile non-tumoral hydrocephalus—A retrospective analysis of 360 cases. *Clinical Neurology and Neurosurgery, 81,* 199-210.

Grellong, B., Vaughan, H., Rotkin, L., Daum, C., Kurtzberg, D., & Lipper, E. (1981, April). Neonatal performance, cognitive and neurologic outcome to 40 months among low birthweight infants. Paper presented at the biennial meeting of the Society for Research in Child Development, Boston.

Griffith, H., & Davidson, M. (1966). Long-term changes in intellect and behavior after hemispherectomy. *Journal of Neurological Psychiatry, 29,* 571-576.

Hebb, D.O. (1942). The effect of early and late brain injury upon test scores and the nature of normal adult intelligence. *Proceedings of the American Philosophical Society, 85,* 275-292.

Karmel, B.Z., & Maisel, E.B. (1975). A neuronal activity model for infant visual attention. In L. Cohen & P. Salapatek (Eds.), *Infant perception: From sensation to cognition* (Vol. 1). New York: Academic Press.

Kenny, P., & Turkewitz, G. (1983, August). Effects of accelerating time of eye opening in rat pups. Paper presented at the meeting of the American Psychological Association, Anaheim.

Kitchen, W.H., Ryan, M.M., Richards, A., McDougall, A.B., Billson, F.A., Keir, E.H., & Naylor, F.D. (1980). A longitudinal study of very low-birthweight infants: An overview of performance at eight years of age. *Developmental Medicine and Child Neurology, 22,* 172-188.

Korner, A.F. (1972). State as variable, as obstacle, and as mediator of stimulation in infant research. *Merrill-Palmer Quarterly, 18,* 77-94.

Kurtzberg, D., Vaughan, H., Daum, C., Grellong, B., Albin, S., & Rotkin, L. (1979). Neurobehavioral performance of low birthweight infants at 40 weeks conceptional age: Comparison with normal full term infants. *Developmental Medicine and Child Neurology, 21,* 590-607.

Lawson, K.R., & Turkewitz, G. (1980). Intersensory functions in newborns: Effect of sound on visual preferences. *Child Development, 51,* 1295-1298.

Lewkowicz, D.J., & Turkewitz, G. (1981). Intersensory interaction in newborns: Modification of visual preferences following exposure to sound. *Child Development, 52,* 280-289.

Lipton, E.L., Steinschneider, A., & Richmond, J.B. (1965). Swaddling, a child practice: Historical, cultural, experimental observations. *Pediatrics, 35,* 521-567.

Maisel, E.B., & Karmel, B.Z. (1978). Contour density and pattern configuration in visual preferences of infants. *Infant Behavior and Development, 1,* 127-140.

McCarvill, S.L., & Karmel, B.Z. (1976). A neural activity interpretation of luminance effects on infant pattern preferences. *Journal of Experimental Child Psychology, 22,* 363-374.

McFie, J. (1961). The effects of hemispherectomy on intellectual functioning in cases of infantile hemiplagia. *Journal of Neurology, Neurosurgery and Psychiatry, 24,* 240-249.

Parmelee, A.H. (1975). Neurophysiological and behavioral organization of preterm infants in the first month of life. *Biological Psychiatry, 10,* 501-512.

Parmelee, A.H., Beckwith, L., Cohen, S.E., & Sigman, M. (1983). Social influences on infants at medical risk for behavioral difficulties. In J. Call, E. Galenson, & R. Tyson (Eds.), *Frontiers of infant psychiatry.* New York: Basic Books.

Piercy, M. (1964). The effects of cerebral lesions on intellectual functioning: A review of current trends. *Annual Review of Psychology, 110,* 310-322.

Prechtl, H.F.R. (1974). The behavioral states of the newborn infant. *Brain Research, 76,* 185-212.

Rie, H.E., & Rie, E.D. (1980). *Handbook of minimal brain dysfunctions. A critical review.* New York: Wiley.

Ruff, H.A., & Turkewitz, G. (1975). Developmental changes in the effectiveness of stimulus intensity on infant visual attention. *Developmental Psychology, 11,* 705-710.

Ruff, H.A., & Turkewitz, G. (1979). Changing role of stimulus intensity as a determinant of infants' attention. *Perceptual and Motor Skills, 48,* 815-826.

Schapiro, S. (1968). Some physiological, biochemical, and behavioral consequences of neonatal hormone administration: Cortisol and thyroxine. *General and Comparative Endocrinology, 10,* 214-228.

Schapiro, S., & Norman, R.J. (1967). Thyroxine: Effects of neonatal administration on maturation, development and behavior. *Science, 155,* 1279-1281.

Schneider, G.C. (1979). Is it really better to have your brain lesion early? A revision of the "Kennard Principle." *Neuropsychologia, 17,* 557-583.

Schneirla, T.C. (1965). Aspects of stimulation and organization in approach/withdrawal processes underlying vertebrate behavioral development. In D.S. Lehrman, R.A. Hinde, & E. Shaw (Eds.), *Advances in the study of behavior* (Vol. 1). New York: Academic Press 1-74.

Sokolov, E.N. (1963). *Perception and the conditioned reflex.* New York: MacMillan.

Sroufe, A.L. (1979). Socioemotional development. In J. Osofsky (Ed.), *Handbook of infant development.* New York: Wiley.

Thoman, E.B. (1981). A biological perspective and a behavioral model for assessment of premature infants. In L.A. Bond & J.M. Joffee (Eds.), *Primary prevention of psychopathology* (Vol. 6). Hanover, N.H.: University Press of New England.

Turkewitz, G., Gardner, J.M., & Lewkowicz, D.J. (1984). Sensory/perceptual functioning during early infancy: The implications of a quantitative basis for responding. In G. Greenberg & E. Tobach (Eds.), *Levels of integration and evolution of behavior.* Hillsdale, N.J.: Lawrence Erlbaum.

Turkewitz, G., Lewkowicz, D.J., & Gardner, J.M. (1983). Determinants of infant perception. In J. Rosenblatt, R.A. Hinde, C. Beer & M. Busnel (Eds.), *Advances in the study of behavior* (Vol. 13). New York: Academic Press.

# Infant Stimulation and Development: Conceptual and Empirical Considerations

Celia A. Brownell, PhD
Mark S. Strauss, PhD

**ABSTRACT.** The last several years have witnessed a growing interest in infant development, and growing concern about infant stimulation. This discussion examines the assumptions about development that underlie the premise that developmental outcomes can be significantly improved by providing early environmental stimulation. Those assumptions include: (a) that infant development is more influenced by environmental factors than by biological/genetic factors; (b) that development is linear and continuous, and that infant development is predictive of later function; (c) that early experiences determine later development; (d) that the normal social environment may be inadequate for optimal development and require improving. Research and theory from developmental psychology provide a different perspective, and a different set of assumptions. Implications for infant intervention and stimulation programs are discussed.

"The child makes the man." Given the tremendous strides in the last fifteen years in our understanding of infant competencies, that old standby has come to carry both more promise and more baggage than ever before. The last several years have seen growing interest in infant development and a corresponding interest in infant stimulation programs. As attested to by the references included in the papers of this volume, literally hundreds of new infant stimulation programs are founded each year. These programs can be divided into two general categories. One group of programs is focused on the infant who is considered at risk for later normal development due to

Celia A. Brownell is Assistant Professor and Mark S. Strauss an Associate Professor in the Department of Psychology at the University of Pittsburgh, Pittsburgh, Pennsylvania 15260.

environmental and/or biological reasons. A second set of programs is concerned with the extent to which the average infant in an adequate environment can be stimulated to develop at a faster rate than normal. Typical of the latter is the Better Baby Institute of Philadelphia which claims to be able to turn *any* infant into an intellectual genius (*Philadelphia Inquirer,* March 15, 1981).

Both categories of programs have emerged as a result of the efforts of individuals who sincerely believe that we can improve the developmental outcome of most children by enhancing their early environmental experiences. Underlying the simple premise that infants will benefit from early extra environmental stimulation are a number of important assumptions about how development occurs, assumptions which must be carefully considered in relation to what is known about human development. Those assumptions include the following: (a) that the early development of an infant is influenced more by the environment than by genetic and biological factors; (b) that development is linear and continuous; (c) that there is a direct and lasting relationship between early experiences and later developmental outcome; and (d) that the normal social environment of the infant may be inadequate for optimal development, and that most infants could benefit from improvements in their naturally occurring social environment.

Such assumptions and intuitions are easily accepted at face value and form the foundation of an implicit and widely-held belief system, one that we believe is misconceived. The following discussion will elaborate our reasoning, based on perspectives from the field of developmental psychology regarding the nature of human development. After all, at its most fundamental level, infant intervention is an attempt to change the course and outcome of development. While that is sometimes a worthy goal, it cannot hope to achieve its ambitions if the models of or assumptions about development on which it is premised are incomplete, oversimplified, or erroneous. Moreover, in many cases, the ambitions themselves may be inappropriate, e.g., given the nature of development, it may be ineffective at best to attempt to stimulate or accelerate development in normal infants raised in normal environments. These are strong, and in some quarters even heretical, statements. Certainly we are not going to advocate doing away with identification and intervention for infants at risk for suboptimal developmental outcome (assuming "suboptimal outcome" can be adequately defined). However, we are arguing that such efforts need to be informed by what little we know about the process of development if they hope to be effective. Accordingly, what we would like to accomplish in this paper is to replace inappropriate assumptions with a more balanced view of development. The discussion will be broken into 4 subsections, each corresponding to a major assumption or set of assumptions characteristic of intervention/stimulation approaches.

## BIOLOGICAL BASES OF DEVELOPMENT

The first assumption to which we will speak constitutes what has often been called "naive environmentalism" (cf. Scarr, 1982). The key components of naive environmentalism are, first, that the environment is the sole determinant of development, and thus by changing selected aspects of the environment the course of development can be changed. That changing the environment may change developmental outcomes is not at issue; what is at issue is whether *every* aspect of development can be so influenced, and how substantial the environmental change must be to produce meaningful and lasting developmental change. A second component, a corollary of the first, is that the developing organism is infinitely malleable. J. B. Watson, of course, produced the classic statement of that position in 1935 with his contention that he could turn any child into any of a number of outcomes, from beggar to lawyer, if he could but control their rearing environments. That tenet is still held today by many.

The flaw in the naive environmentalism assumption is that it fails to recognize the inherently biological nature of development. We do not intend to raise the old spectre of nature-nurture arguments here: development is the result of continuous, dynamic interaction between the organism's biology and the organism's environment. Nature and nurture are mutually interdependent. That is to say, among other things, that the biological influences on development do not begin and end at conception, but are a major, enduring source of influence on the *process* of development. We will identify three levels at which biological influences are relevant to development: (1) species patterns in development; (2) the genetics of behavior and development; and (3) biological development of the central nervous system.

*Species patterns.* It is no coincidence that sensorimotor development comprises the first 24-36 months of every normal child's life, or that every normal child acquires a first language within the first

3-5 years of life, or that puberty has its onset between 11 and 15 years for every child. The universal pattern of human development is as much a product of evolution as is human language, upright posture, or the opposable thumb. It is not inappropriate to speak of a species "program" for development. For our purposes it is important to consider two aspects of that program: which developments it comprises, and why; and what role the environment plays in producing outcomes from the program.

Life carries with it the potential for incredible variety. The genes that are the foundation of life can assort, mutate, and recombine into innumerable constellations, some viable, some not. Humans, for example, possess 46 chromosomes, each of which carries perhaps 10,000 genes; the number of possible permutations of those half million genes is awesome. Given that each new human is a wholly new and unique genotype,[1] and given the vast potential for genetic variability, how is it that human phenotypes[2] are essentially alike? Similarly, given the variety of normal human environments in which all of those unique genotypes develop, how is it that there are species-specific, human universals in behavior and development? That is, how is it that we all turn out to look, behave, and develop like humans, given the genetic differences among us? Behavior geneticists and embryologists have posited a mechanism for restricting phenotypic variability while preserving genotypic variability. Genetic variability is essential to evolution. If each individual were genetically and phenotypically identical, fluctuations in the environment could produce mass extinction. With genetic variability, the likelihood exists that some individuals will possess the means for adaptation to a changed environment. But phenotypic restriction is also necessary for survival: the frog and the princess could not exploit the same niche, nor reproduce. This mechanism has been termed *canalization* (Waddington, 1962).

Compelling illustrations of this phenomenon are provided by embryologists who have studied, and manipulated genetically, the "self-righting" tendencies of organisms during development following insult to the growing system. For example, when a developing embryo is subjected to some adverse, environmental influence the degree to which it is affected during later growth, producing an abnormal outcome, can be varied by selective breeding (Waddington, 1966). The conclusion is that the developing system has a built-in, genetically based tendency to resist deflection by external forces from a predetermined developmental pathway. Hence, these paths are said to be "canalized." This canalization restricts the variability of phenotypes to one or a few developmental outcomes within the species-typical range of environments. Note that this concept includes as a central and necessary component the role of the environment. The environment is necessary for the expression of the genotype as phenotype, but the environment is not all-powerful in determining the final form of the phenotype; part of that determination lies with the species program.

Every species-universal characteristic, whether physiological or behavioral, is presumed to follow one of these canalized growth paths. Thus, different genotypes and/or different environments tend to produce similar phenotypes. This is not to say that development cannot be altered by alterations in the environment. Certainly it can be, and often is. But those environmental insults that produce drastic disruptions in outcome are themselves drastic, and far outside the range of normal environmental variation for the species. Moreover, not every developmental pathway is equally strongly canalized; some aspects of development are more easily deflected by environmental variation than others. Thus, the course of language acquisition appears to be highly canalized: it requires a grossly inadequate linguistic environment to deflect the sequence of normal language development and to produce an abnormal outcome; normal children acquire a first language at remarkably similar ages in remarkably similar sequences within a vast range of language learning environments. For development, all of those environments are functionally equivalent. Childhood IQ, however, as measured by standardized tests, is not so highly canalized. Fluctuations within the range of normal environments produce different outcomes; the developmental pathways here are not so resistant to deflection by "the winds of environmental change," and different environments are not functionally equivalent for producing developmental outcome.

It appears that those characteristics which have been most necessary to survival and reproduction are those that are most strongly canalized, thus the most buffered against deviation due to environmental variations. In infancy, such characteristics must include at least the propensity to form a primary attachment to a caregiver (Bowlby, 1969), basic cognitive developmental competencies (Piaget, 1952), and a first language (Brown, 1973). They may also include higher-order social abilities and/or cognitive abilities. However, they almost certainly do not include abilities such as reading, arithmetic, playing a musical instrument, reciting poetry, or the relatively complex world knowledge on which such advanced skills are based.

Let us note again that the point is not that canalized aspects of development "simply mature," in the absence of environmental input. Rather, the point is that the primary developments characteristic of infancy find the necessary degree of environmental support and quality of input within the normal range of human environments. Because all normal infants raised within the range of normal environments will eventually acquire all the major, foundational competencies of human infancy from object permanence to social interaction skills to language, despite individual differences in the rates of such acquisitions, we have no grounds for assuming that acceleration of those acquisitions will make a difference in the long run. Indeed, as will be discussed later, there is little predictability from infancy to later childhood or adolescent functioning.

The conclusions from these points are that the infant's environment is not the sole determinant, or even the primary determinant of developmental outcome; that the infant is not infinitely malleable; that the "species program" seems to provide strong buffers against adverse developmental consequences from variations in early environments. Hence, one would expect limits in the extent to which stimulation programs can affect the normal course of development, especially for those early abilities which are highly canalized.

## Genetics of Development

We have been discussing the influence of the genotype on development at the species level. What about genotypes at the level of the individual? While an individual's genotype may be canalized for species-specific and species-universal patterns of development, it is still unique: what does the uniqueness confer on the individual's development? Among other things, it should specify different and unique responses for each individual to a given environment. Again, note that we are not suggesting genetic determination of developmental outcomes, rather we are discussing the nature of gene-environment transactions that constitute the *process* of development.

Behavior geneticists (cf. Scarr & Kidd, 1983) have given us the concept of *reaction range* to characterize one of the relationships between an individual's genotype and the phenotypic outcome due to unique gene-environment transactions. Reaction range embodies the fact that an individual possesses a range of potential developmental outcomes from a single genotype. That range of outcomes corresponds to the range of environments in which the individual might develop. Thus, an infant's developmental outcome is partly a function of her genotype which specifies the range of reaction, and partly a function of the environment in which that genotype becomes expressed. For example, although variations in socioeconomic status do not produce differences in a child's mastery of basic syntactic rules, they often do produce differences in vocabulary and pre-reading skills. Similarly, in the same environment different children with different genotypes will both acquire basic syntax at the same level of mastery, but they may well not acquire equivalent pre-reading or reading skills. In other words, different environments produce variations in developmental outcome, but genotypes also affect the degree in which environmental influences are able to produce variation.

A fine example of the concept of reaction range has been provided by a study of IQ in adopted children who were raised in the "environment of the IQ test" (Scarr & Weinberg, 1976). To summarize very briefly, these authors followed the progress of a large number of children adopted into advantaged white middle- or upper-middle-class homes. Many of these children were Black, Native American, or Vietnamese. On the basis of information about the children's biological parents, their projected IQ's would have been expected to be subnormal had they remained with their biological parents. However, their IQ's were, in fact, substantially above normal. While the relationship of the children's IQ was higher to biological than to adoptive parents, the absolute level of their IQ's was a function of their changed, adoptive environments. Thus, each child was born with a large range of potential developmental outcomes for IQ, from low to high. But, by the same token, each child's potential was different from the next child's. In other words, not all children are born potential geniuses; but for some aspects of development, IQ included, each child is born with a range of possible outcomes and each child's particular outcome within that range will depend on characteristics of the environment. Thus, the effects of the environment on development are modified or qualified by the child's individual genotype. While the infant possesses a range of possible developmental outcomes, there remain limits on these outcomes; however the infant is not somehow "at the mercy" of his

genes. Both genes and environment act in concert, over developmental time, to produce species-general phenotypes as well as
unique, individual patterns within that larger pattern.

## Biological Development of the Central Nervous System

Another aspect of the naive environmentalism assumption is that
external stimulation can increase the rate at which the cerebral cortex develops, i.e., that appropriate stimulation can "speed-up the
biological clock" of the brain. The empirical evidence suggests that
this assumption is incorrect. In this section we will discuss two main
avenues of research addressed to this question.

The human brain is composed of approximately 10 billion individual neurons[3] all of which are interconnected and continuously
"communicating" with each other. It is this vast network of interconnected neurons which provides the "hardware" or basis for all
intellectual functioning. While we are born with all of the neurons
we will ever have in life, they undergo extensive development
through childhood, particularly during the first two years of life.
This is especially true of the largest area of the brain, the cerebral
cortex, which is the center of all higher intellectual functions including our ability to speak, or to ponder abstract concepts such as love
and honesty. More specifically, extensive anatomical study of the
infant's cerebral cortex has shown that the dendrites of a neuron (the
part of a neuron that interconnect with other neurons) continue to
develop sub-branches so that over the first two years of life the
brain's communication network becomes increasingly complex.
Additionally, the neurons (or axons) of the cerebral cortex in adults
have a type of coating or insulation known as the myelin sheath.
This coating allows the neuron to transmit impulses at a much faster
rate than an unmyelinated neuron. In comparison to the mature cerebral cortex, many of the neurons in the newborn's brain are unmyelinated, and this myelinization process occurs at a very rapid pace
during the first two years (Conel, 1939, 1941, 1947, 1951, 1959).
Thus at birth, the "hardware" of the human's brain is still extremely underdeveloped.

One major area of research dealing with brain development has
been conducted on lower animals (usually rats) who are raised in
either deprived or enriched environments. In these studies, one
group of rats is raised in ordinary lab cages which provide very little
environmental stimulation (i.e., deprived). A second group of rats is

raised in a rich and complex environment, e.g., a large cage containing other rats and a number of toys and objects which can be explored (i.e., enriched). To measure the effects of these two environments on development, researchers typically look for differences in the brains of the two groups, and the extent to which they differ on various measures of "intelligence" such as learning to run through a maze. In general, these studies have demonstrated that when rats are raised in an enriched environment, their brains develop more dendritic branches and they solve mazes better than rats who are raised in deprived environments (e.g., Greenough, 1975, 1979; Rosenzweig, Bennett, & Diamond, 1972).

Can it be inferred from these studies that human infants who are in stimulation programs will demonstrate faster or increased biological development of the brain and higher levels of intelligence? First it must be recognized that the animals in the above experiments were being reared in two extremely different environments 24 hours a day. This was necessary since the differences found between the two groups of rats are typically quite small and would probably not emerge under less extreme conditions. Compare this to the average infant program which provides a relatively small increase in stimulation over what is already a normal environment, and for only a few hours out of the day. While the results of the animal research clearly indicate that under extreme conditions the environment can have an effect on the development of the brain, it is highly unlikely that comparable results would be gained from the minimal increase in stimulation that occurs from the typical program for infants. Indeed, a comparable study on human infants would require that a group of babies be raised in an isolated, sound-proof room devoid of toys or other subjects ("deprived"), and then compared to infants raised in normal environments ("enriched"). Under such conditions, ethically unthinkable, it would not be surprising to find developmental differences. Fortunately, such deprived conditions do not correspond to any but the most severely neglectful of human environments.

Second, it must be recognized that rats develop at a much faster rate than humans—rats reach adult maturity by approximately one month of age. Thus animal stimulation studies look at the effects of different environments over essentially the entire "childhood" of the animal. In comparison, most infant stimulation programs cover only a small portion of an extended, 12 to 15 year childhood. Thus, while the research being conducted with animals raised in different environments is of scientific import and interest, it lends little support to the notion that human infant stimulation will speed up the course of biological development.

A second area of research to consider with respect to whether it is possible to enhance the development of the central nervous system through stimulation is research which has been conducted with premature infants. Most human births in the United States occur at 38-40 weeks after conception. However, approximately 10 to 15 percent of the infants in this country are born after a shorter gestational period, with approximately 7 percent of the infants being born prior to 37 weeks of gestation (Keller, 1981). Over the last 10 to 15 years there has been increasingly concern with the development of these premature infants, in particular whether they are at risk for later problems. These studies also provide a natural way to study the effects of environmental stimulation on development. If one compares two infants, both of whom are 4 months old with respect to postnatal age (age from birth), but where one of the infants was actually born 1 month prematurely, it is apparent that the premature infant is actually one month younger than the full-term infant with respect to conceptional age (the age from conception). But this younger, premature baby has had 4 months' postnatal experience and thus has the "advantage" of an extra month of extrauterine environmental stimulation. The question then arises as to whether these two infants are comparable in their developmental levels as a result of equivalent amounts of experience, or whether the premature infant is one month behind as a result of his younger conceptional age.

Several aspects of development have been compared in full-term and premature infants. Investigators have looked at the course of brain development by use of a computer averaged EEG known as an Evoked Potential (e.g., Rose, 1981). Similarly, a number of studies have compared premature and full-term infants with respect to auditory development (e.g., Parmelee, 1981), visual development (e.g., Dobson, Mayer, & Lee, 1980) and visual recognition memory (e.g., Fantz & Miranda, 1927; Rose, Gottfried, & Bridge, 1979). The overwhelming conclusion of this research is that development of basic sensory processes and early cognitive skills such as recognition memory and visual pattern preferences is based on physiological maturation and that the longer period of environmental stimulation has essentially no effect. In other words, when one compares the sensory or cognitive abilities of, for example, two

4 month old infants, one of whom was born a month prematurely, the premature infant is typically one month behind the full-term infant in development, despite the fact that the premature infant has had an equal amount of exposure to the external environment.

In summary, no researcher would argue against the idea that the environment can have a dramatic impact on the physiological maturation of the central nervous system. This is especially clear when the environment is particularly impoverished (e.g., an animal raised blindfolded would unquestionably suffer deterioration of the parts of the brain concerned with vision). However, it is much less clear that minor differences in a normal environment, especially during the first year or two, have any impact on the development of the brain. Indeed, at this point, existing research would suggest that infants raised in essentially normal environments would gain no benefits with respect to central nervous system maturation as a result of increased early stimulation. While the above would argue against the notion that for normal infants in normal environments, stimulation programs would have a dramatic effect on brain growth, this implication is less clear for infants who have some type of physical damage to the brain. At present, the extent to which environmental stimulation can affect the brain's ability to "overcome" such damage is unknown and direct research on this issue is imperative.

## DEVELOPMENTAL DISCONTINUITY

A second pervasive assumption which needs to be addressed is that development inherently and necessarily happens in a linear, continuous manner. It is commonly held by both professionals and nonprofessionals alike that infant functioning should be directly predictive of childhood functioning: the smart infant becomes the smart child; the active infant becomes the active child; the sociable infant becomes the sociable child. More generally, it is assumed that the precocious infant will be similarly accelerated in childhood, and, conversely, that the slow infant will be behind as a child.

The problems with this assumption are both empirical and conceptual: there appear to be few such continuities from infancy to childhood, even when investigators set out explicitly to look for them; nor is it altogether clear whether we should expect such continuities. One issue, of course, is what level of analysis is appropriate in the search for developmental continuity (cf. Sroufe, 1979).

We do not wish to embroil this discussion in that or related issues, although it should be recognized that they ultimately must be raised if questions about developmental continuity are to be resolved. Our aim here is first to point up the empirical difficulties with the developmental continuity assumption at the level at which it is commonly instantiated in infant intervention/stimulation programs. We will also briefly discuss the conceptual issue of whether development, in principle, should be expected to exhibit continuities from infancy to childhood at the customary level of analysis. Our discussion of developmental continuity and predictability will be limited to the level of analysis and the areas of functioning that are the focus of infant programs. The level of analysis to which we are referring is, of course, the usual battery of outcome measures meant to evaluate the developmental status of the infant or child. These typically include standardized intelligence tests such as the Bayley Scales of Infant Development or the WISC-R, standardized tests of receptive and/or productive language function, and sometimes a global measure of social skill. The question, then, is whether individual differences on some discrete outcome measure (or set of measures) remain stable from infancy to childhood.

The fact is that few investigations using such measures have found evidence that behavior and development during the first 24 months of life predicts to functioning in later childhood, although many such investigations have been mounted (cf. Beckwith, 1979; Kopp & McCall, 1982; McCall, 1979, 1981; Sameroff, 1976; Shaffer & Dunn, 1979). This seems to hold for studies of mental development, language development, and social/emotional development.

The data on mental development will serve as a good illustration. Individual differences on IQ tests remain quite stable after middle childhood, more so than most other behavioral characteristics (McCall, 1979). Because of our propensity to view IQ as a constant part of an individual's make-up, that probably comes as no surprise. But by the same reasoning, we would expect this characteristic of "intelligence" to have been the child's from birth, and to have been revealed in all of the child's performances during development. Yet longitudinal studies of intellectual functioning have revealed correlations of only .06 to .32 for IQ scores between infancy and middle to late childhood (McCall, 1979). That contrasts with correlations as high as .80 to .90 between middle and late childhood (Kopp & McCall, 1982). In other words, while there is a relatively strong relationship in IQ scores between middle and late childhood, almost no relationship exists between infancy and middle to late childhood. In the Fels longitudinal sample, McCall (1973) reported that the average change in IQ between 2-1/2 and 17 years was 28.5 points (potentially, the difference between "gifted" and "retarded"), and a number of individuals shifted as much as 40 points. Even within infancy, IQ scores are relatively unstable, showing only moderate correlations over as little time as a few months during the first 2 years of life. Moreover, these patterns are remarkably similar for handicapped or biologically at-risk infants (Kopp & McCall, 1982).

What are the reasons for this instability of individual differences in infancy, and the lack of predictability from infancy to childhood? There certainly are psychometric variables such as test-retest reliability that may enter into the problem. But McCall (1979) has argued that such effects are probably minimal. The explanation for these patterns is more often a variant of the axiom "development is change." Specifically, most developmental psychologists have argued that infancy constitutes a unique and qualitatively different period of psychological functioning than does later childhood (e.g., McCall, 1981; Piaget, 1952; Scarr-Salapatek, 1976). Because of the major developmental reorganization that occurs around 24 months, permitting the emergence of a symbol system (e.g., language) and much more complex cognitive and social functioning, many authors hold that predictability from infancy should not be expected. Indeed, Scarr-Salapatek (1976) has argued that infant intelligence is a "primate theme," and that sensorimotor level abilities are essentially unrelated to subsequent intellectual abilities, except of course as the foundation on which later abilities must be constructed. But, she argues, because sensorimotor intelligence will develop in all species-members raised in a species-typical environment, it is fruitless to expect predictability to the later intellectual functioning which is uniquely human, more recently evolved, and entails a wholly different set of competencies.

The obvious conclusion here is that we cannot assume that infant characteristics will remain stable and will come to characterize the child, adolescent or adult. Concretely, that means that except for clear cases of extensive CNS damage, we cannot conclude that the slow infant will necessarily grow up to become the slow child. While that is a hopeful statement for intervention attempts because it attests to developmental plasticity, it is simultaneously and equally importantly a statement conveying caution—if we can't accurately predict which infants will be developmentally delayed as children on the basis of their functioning during infancy, it makes early intervention/stimulation substantially more difficult to justify, particularly for low-risk infants. It also suggests that some of the positive outcomes of early intervention may be artifacts of low predictability.

## IMPERMANENCE OF EARLY EXPERIENCE EFFECTS

The third focus of our discussion centers on the "early experience" assumption. Because this issue has been presented in detail elsewhere in this volume (Ramey), we will only briefly address it here. The early experience assumption in its most general form takes as a given that the child's early encounters with the environment carry proportionately more weight for developmental outcome than similar experiences later. Hence the increasingly strong emphasis on earlier and earlier interventions. There are two corollaries of this assumption. One can be termed the "inoculation" position, and holds that the positive effects of early experience should be maintained in subsequent functioning. The idea is that beneficial early experiences inoculate the child, in a sense, against later "blows" that the environment may deliver to development. The second is the "devastation" position, and emphasizes the long-term negative consequences of suboptimal or depriving early environmental conditions, even if such deprivation is temporary.

The early experience assumption is engrained in the very fabric of much of developmental psychology, and is not unique to intervention/stimulation arguments. It has a long history not only in Western thought (Kagan, 1978) but also in the foundational theoretical systems of developmental psychology. It has received support from animal work (e.g., Lorenz, 1935; Scott & Fuller, 1962; Rosenblatt & Lehrmann, 1963), and later studies of institutionalized children (Bowlby, 1951) lent additional credibility to generalizations from animals to humans. This assumption currently commands widespread popular support in the form of mother-infant "bonding," held to occur in the first few minutes after birth and presumed to be crucial to subsequent high-quality mother-infant interaction (Klaus & Kennell, 1976).

However, despite its historical force, intuitive appeal, popular support, and analogues in the animal literature, the early experience position has recently come under increasing scrutiny and criticism by mainstream developmental psychologists. The reasons for the criticism are varied. Perhaps the most convincing, however, is the growing amount of data which fail to support it. The first hint of such failure came from the now widely known finding that compensatory education programs, while producing sometimes remarkable gains for children during their tenure, did not produce long term gains (see Ramey, this volume). Indeed, once having graduated from such programs, children begin to exhibit a progressive and steady decline until, after a few years, they become indistinguishable from their counterparts who did not have such remedial early experience. On the other side of the coin, numerous investigators have found recovery from poor early experience once the child's depriving environment is replaced with an adequate one (e.g., Kagan & Klein, 1973; Sameroff & Chandler, 1975; Skeels, 1966). Even the apparently robust findings of irreversible devastation due to prolonged deprivation in Harlow's rhesus macaques have now been shown to be reversible when the environment is appropriately altered (Novak & Harlow, 1975). In a similar vein, the Clarkes (Clarke & Clarke, 1976) have amassed impressive evidence showing that the effects of severe deprivation and/or abuse of human children in their early years, which produced massive behavioral and intellectual retardation, can also be reversed when the children are transferred into normal environments. Although such results are surprising to the early experience assumption, they are predictable from a canalization position, which recognizes the strong self-righting tendencies of the organism and buffering against permanent deviation from the developmental trajectory.

The conclusion to be drawn from these sorts of findings is not that early experience is unimportant for development. Rather, the implications are first that a child's earliest experiences do not necessarily carry more weight for developmental outcome than do later experiences, but that the quality of experience at every age is important to outcome, and second, that *cumulative* experience, good or bad, is more important than the absolute timing of experience. In other words, later experiences and later development extend and build on earlier environmental input and developmental foundations. *Early* good or poor experiences will not alone provide definitive developmental outcomes if subsequent environments change, but *cumulative* good or poor experiences can and do. Early experience is but one factor in a much larger system of dynamic, interacting factors over the whole of development. And it is not a proportionately more important one. Rather, experiences at all periods of development are critical to outcome.

## SOCIAL FOUNDATIONS OF DEVELOPMENT

That development has a social as well as a biological foundation is hardly news to an intervention/stimulation perspective. What we would like to consider here, quite briefly, is the supposition that the infant's normal, everyday social environment must be "beefed up" to provide optimal levels of stimulation or cognitive support for development. The alternative position derives from several of the previous points, particularly from the concept of canalization. That position is that the normal range of human social environments (and that range is quite broad, not restricted to the norm for white, middle class families) provides the necessary support for normal development in normal infants. We, of course, do not include overtly neglecting or abusive parents in our implicit definition of "normal range." The reasoning is that human development is a function of evolution, and that human development and evolution have occurred in a social context (cf. Scarr-Salapatek, 1976). In other words, infancy has evolved in a network of social relations characteristic of our species—the "environment of evolutionary adaptedness" has been and remains predominantly a *social* environment.

What are the implications? At the broadest level, one implication is that the natural, unintervened transactions between the infant and a responsive social environment will be co-adapted to produce normal outcome. Those co-adaptations take several, universal forms. First, the social world provides perceptual and cognitive stimulation as well as social. It is probably no accident that the human face possesses just those stimulus characteristics that are salient and attractive to the neonate (Cohen, DeLoache, & Strauss, 1979), and that because of the incentives to the parent for social interaction, those stimulus characteristics are presented often and in the optimal visual space for the newborn. Another complex of co-adaptations can be seen in the infant's propensity to respond to contingent stimulation (Watson, 1979) and the social environment's tendency to respond contingently to the infant (Stern, 1977). Similar co-adaptation between the developing infant and the social environment can be shown to exist for the infant's tendency to respond to moderate discrepancy or novelty (Kagan, 1979), for information necessary to learn about object (person) permanence, spatial and temporal relations, causation, and so forth. The social environment is a rich and changing source of stimulation and information for the infant, co-adapted with the infant's developmental competencies and requirements. Moreover, parents explicitly control and adapt the amount and timing of social stimulation, as well as its level of complexity to keep pace with the infant's current developmental level and to challenge the infant to move ahead (e.g., Crawley et al., 1978; Gustafson et al., 1979).

Although to many, particularly to parents, this line of reasoning and these sorts of observations seems intuitively obvious, they are often ignored in the press to enhance the normal environments of many babies in order to stimulate and accelerate their development. To the extent that the concern for stimulation may disrupt the baby's normal social environment, and insofar as we know of no research documenting that acceleration of infant development produces lasting positive consequences, early stimulation in lieu of the ordinary but rich social involvement of parents and infants seems questionable.

Our primary point is that infant development by nature is embedded in a complex social environment; that web of social involvements serves multiple necessary functions for the growing infant, and is intricately tied up with and co-adapted with the biological bases of development. Further, parents are also part of this network of co-adaptations—parenting has evolved to optimize the development of offspring. Hence for most parents, parent-infant social involvement is by nature adapted to the needs of the infant.

## SUMMARY AND CONCLUSIONS

Most individuals involved with implementing infant stimulation programs are concerned with research that helps them decide exactly what types of interventions or procedures will be most effective in enhancing the child's subsequent development. Rarely is thought given to the more basic questions of whether infant stimulation works and what assumptions must underlie a belief in the efficacy of early stimulation programs. In this paper we have attempted to raise, to discuss, and to put into a *developmental* perspective those assumptions.

Briefly, we have suggested that:

1. Research from the fields of genetics and developmental psychobiology appears to indicate that while particularly impoverished environments can have a dramatic influence on the physiological maturation of the central nervous system, most differences in nor-

mal environments, especially during the first year or two, probably have little, if any, long term impact on development of the brain or behavior. That is because there are strong genetic and biological influences operating during the infancy period which "guarantee" that infants will develop necessary sensorimotor and social skills even in the face of substantial variations in the environment. Indeed, most mildly compromised infants demonstrate remarkable catch-up growth without additional stimulation, as the concept of canalization would predict. Thus, it is unlikely that broad-based stimulation programs (which typically represent a minor variation in an already normal environment) will have a major or longlasting impact on early development. Naturally, an infant being raised in an extremely abnormal environment would be expected to benefit from programs which attempted to correct such problems. Similarly, it is difficult to predict what impact stimulation might have on infants with clear evidence of brain damage. Such handicapped infants may not possess the biological mechanisms needed to interact effectively with the "average" environment and thus may need skill-specific guidance or extra stimulation. Unfortunately, at this point there is little research to indicate exactly what types of stimulation might be appropriate for these brain-damaged infants.

2. It cannot be assumed that infant characteristics will remain stable and thus come to characterize the child, adolescent or adult. Indeed, the preponderance of research has indicated that, with the exception of cases in which the infant has extensive central nervous system damage, measures of infant functioning and development do not predict later development. This fact has two important implications. First, if we are not able to predict accurately which infants will be developmentally delayed as children on the basis of their functioning during infancy, it is difficult to justify early intervention or stimulation for low-risk or normal infants who do not evidence clear biological deficits. Second, it is possible that the reported positive outcomes of some early intervention programs may be artifacts of this low predictability.

3. Development is a cumulative process. Early good or poor experiences will not alone provide predictable developmental outcome if subsequent environments change, but cumulative good or poor experiences can and do. This principle is especially important if prevention of poor outcome, rather than "treatment," is the priority. The "inoculation" form of the early experience assumption does not hold up under scrutiny. For any intervention/stimulation pro-

gram to be effective, it is vital that it not focus on a single period of development. Rather, it will have to be carried forward through childhood if relatively more permanent effects are to emerge.

4. Most parents naturally provide their infants with a social environment which is a rich and changing source of stimulation. Moreover, parents explicitly control and adapt the amount and timing of stimulation, as well as its level of complexity to keep pace with the infant's current developmental level and to challenge the infant to move ahead. Thus, most infants develop in what is probably already an "ideal" environment, one that is especially tailored to their cognitive, perceptual, and social development needs. Indeed, to the extent that a stimulation program disrupts this natural environment, it may even be harmful.

However, some mildly compromised infants and even some uncompromised infants will fail to develop optimally. These infants are categorized as being at risk because of suboptimal rearing environments. Two points are relevant here. First, although it is difficult to disentangle issues of culture-bound definitions of optimality from a discussion of these children's outcomes, we can discuss the influences on development at a more abstract level. On the basis of previous points, we can expect such infants eventually to accomplish the basic and universal competencies of infancy, albeit at a slower rate perhaps. However, later childhood academic skills, social competence, achievement motivation, self-concept, and so forth may be affected: these are presumably less canalized and more open to environmental influence. Given the discussion above, it is not at all evident that infant stimulation will directly or indirectly affect these later-developing characteristics. Rather, direct intervention after infancy, specific to whatever characteristics are deemed important for optimal outcome would seem both more appropriate and more effective.

Second, one would expect that stimulation programs would be effective when focused on helping parents who are not able to interact with their infants in a natural and comfortable manner. Such situations might arise as a result of parental personal or interpersonal problems (e.g., extreme depression), or parental immaturity (e.g., teenage parents), or parental inability to cope with an infant born with some type of handicap. In such cases, parental intervention or support would probably have greater impact than stimulation focused on the infant alone.

At the most general level, the above considerations have been incorporated into a model of development come to be known as the "transactional" model. This model takes into account a changing organism, a changing environment, and the mutual, reciprocal, and continuous effects of these on one another over time. Development is construed as a constructive process on the part of an active, thinking child who selects, interprets and structures his environment as a function of current competencies. The child is continuously changing due to her developmental program—e.g., at 6-8 weeks she responds with a social smile for the first time and begins to coo and babble; at 8-10 months she begins to take initiative in social interactions, shows clear preference for caregivers, and begins to exhibit the beginnings of problem-solving skills. And the changing child requires changing adaptations from the environment, particularly the social environment. But that environment is also changing. Hence the child is part of a *system*—a co-adapted set of changes that are interdependent, mutually influencing one another over time. There is no single, unidirectional cause of outcome: Neither the child nor the child's environment alone is predictive of developmental outcome.

## NOTES

1. Genotype: an individual's genetic make-up.
2. Phenotype: an individual's observable characteristics, including anatomical and physical features as well as behavior.
3. Neuron: part of the nervous system that transmits impulses.

## REFERENCES

Beckwith, L. (1979). Prediction of emotional and social behavior. In J. Osofsky (Ed.), *Handbook of Infant Development.* New York: John Wiley & Sons.

Bowlby, J. (1969). *Attachment.* New York: Basic Books.

Bowlby, J. (1951). *Maternal care and mental health.* Geneva: WHO Monographs.

Brown, R. (1973). *A first language: The early stages.* Massachusetts: Harvard University Press.

Clarke, A., & Clarke, A. (1976). *Early experience: Myth and evidence.* New York: Free Press.

Conel, J. L. (1939-1959). *The postnatal development of the human cerebral cortex,* vols. 1-6. Cambridge, Mass.: Harvard University Press.

Crawley, S., Rogers, P., Friedman, S., Lacobbo, M., Criticos, A., Richardson, L., & Thompson, M. (1978). Developmental changes in the structure of mother-infant play. *Developmental Psychology, 14,* 30-36.

Dobson, V., Mayer, D. L., & Lee, C. P. (1980). Visual acuity screening of preterm infants. *Invest. Opthal. Vis. Sci., 19,* 1498-1505.

Fantz, R. L., & Miranda, S. B. (1977). Visual processing in newborn, preterm, and mentally high-risk infants. In L. Gluck (Ed.), *Intrauterine asphyxia and developing fetal brain.* Chicago: Year Book Medical Publishers.

Greenough, W. T. (1975). Experiential modification of the developing brain. *American Scientist, 63,* 37-46.

Greenough, W. T., Juraska, J. M., & Volkmar, F. R. (1979). Maze training effects on dendritic branching in occipital cortex of adult rats. *Behavioral and Neural Biology, 26,* 287-297.

Gustafson, G., Green, J., & West, M. (1979). The infant's changing role in mother-infant games: The growth of social skills. *Infant Behavior and Development, 2,* 301-308.

Kagan, J., & Klein, R. (1973). Cross-cultural perspectives on early development. *American Psychologist, 28,* 947-961.

Kagan, J. (1979). Structure and process in the human infant: The ontogeny of mental representation. In M. Bornstein and W. Kessen (Eds.), *Psychological development from infancy: Image to intention.* Hillsdale, N.J.: L. Erlbaum.

Keller, C. A. (1981). Epidemiological characteristics of preterm births. In S. L. Friedman and M. Sigman (Eds.), *Preterm birth and psychological development.* New York: Academic Press, 1981.

Klaus, M., & Kennell, J. (1976). *Maternal-infant bonding.* St. Louis: C. V. Mosby.

Kopp, C., & McCall, R. (1982). Predicting later mental performance for normal, at-risk and handicapped infants. In P. Baltes and O. Brim (Eds.), *Life-span development and behavior, vol. 4.* New York: Academic Press.

Lorenz, K. (1935). Der Kumpen in der Unwelt des Vogels. *Journal of Ornithology, 79;* translated in R. Martin (Ed.), *Studies in Animal and Human Behavior.* Cambridge, Mass.: Harvard University Press.

McCall, R. (1979). The development of intellectual functioning in infancy and the prediction of later IQ. In J. Osofsky (Ed.), *Handbook of Infant Development.* New York: John Wiley & Sons.

McCall, R. (1981). Nature-nurture and the two realms of developmental psychology: A proposed integration with respect to mental development. *Child Development, 52,* 1-12.

Novak, M., & Harlow, H. (1975). Social recovery of monkeys isolated for the first year of life. *Developmental Psychology, 11,* 453-465.

Parmelee, A. H. (1981). Auditory function and neurological maturation in preterm infants. In S. F. Friedman and M. Sigman (Eds.), *Preterm birth and psychological development.* New York: Academic Press.

Piaget, J. (1952). *The origins of intelligence in children.* New York: International University Press.

Rose, G. H. (1981). Animal studies in developmental psychobiology: Commentary in method, theory, and human implications. In S. L. Friedman and M. Sigman (Eds.), *Preterm birth and psychological development.* New York: Academic Press.

Rose, S. A., Gottfried, A. W., & Bridger, W. H. Effects of haptic cues on visual recognition memory in fullterm and preterm infants. *Infant Behavior and Development, 2,* 55-67.

Rosenblatt, J., & Lehrman, D. (1963). Maternal behavior in the laboratory rat. In H. Rheingold (Ed.), *Maternal behavior in mammals.* New York: John Wiley & Sons.

Rosenzweig, M. R., Bennet, E. L., & Diamond, M. C. (1972). Chemical and anatomical plasticity of the brain: Replications and extensions. In J. Gaito (Ed.), *Macro-molecules and behavior,* 2nd edition. New York: Appleton-Century-Crofts.

Sameroff, A. (1976). Early influences on development: Fact or fancy? *Merrill-Palmer Quarterly, 21,* 267-294.

Sameroff, A., & Chandler, M. (1975). Reproductive risk and the continuum of caretaking casualty. In F. Horowitz (Ed.), *Review of Child Development Research,* vol. 4. Chicago: University of Chicago Press.

Scarr, S. (1982). On quantifying the intended effects of interventions: A proposed theory of the environment. In L. Bond and J. Joffe (Eds.), *Facilitating infant and early childhood development.* New Hampshire: University Press of New England.

Scarr, S., & Kidd, K. (1983). Developmental behavior genetics. In P. Mussen (Ed.), *Handbook of Child Psychology,* 4th edition. New York: John Wiley & Sons.

Scarr, S., & Weinberg, R. (1976). IQ test performance of black children adopted by white families. *American Psychologist, 31,* 726-739.

Scarr-Salapatek, S. (1976). An evolutionary perspective on infant intelligence. In M. Lewis (Ed.), *Origins of intelligence.* New York: Plenum.

Scott, J. (1962). Critical periods in behavioral development. *Science, 138,* 949-958.

Shaffer, D., & Dunn, J. (Eds.). (1979). *The first year of life: Psychological and medical implications of early experience.* Chichester: John Wiley & Sons.

Skeels, H. (1966). Adult status of children with contrasting early life experiences. *Monographs of the Society for Research in Child Development, 31*(no.3).

Sroufe, L. A. (1979). The coherence of individual development: Early care, attachment and subsequent developmental issues. *American Psychologist, 34,* 834-841.

Stern, D. (1977). *The first relationship.* Cambridge, Mass.: Harvard University Press.

Waddington, C. H. (1962). *New patterns in genetics and development.* New York: Columbia University Press.

Waddington, C. H. (1966). *Principles of development and differentiation.* London: Macmillan.

Watson, J. B. (1928). *Psychological care of the infant and child.* New York: Norton.

Watson, J. S. (1979). Perception of contingency as a determinant of social responsiveness. In E. Thoman (Ed.), *Origins of the infant's social responsiveness.* Hillsdale, N.J.: L. Erlbaum.

*Part IV*

*COMMENTARY*

# A Commentary on Infant Stimulation and Intervention

Mark S. Strauss, PhD
Celia A. Brownell, PhD

The hope of any editor when putting together a journal or book which is intended to address a single topic is that the papers will focus on issues and thus allow for the emergence of common themes. While this is a noble goal, in practice such agreement rarely occurs. Thus, editors seek an individual who will find the "common threads" and write a commentary which makes diverse papers sound similar. Of course, this is often an impossible task and the "threads" which emerge usually appear to be synthetic and rather weak. Fortunately, the individual writing the commentary has an easy solution to this problem; he or she can simply write individual summaries of each of the papers and then suggest to the reader that the papers do in fact address common issues and that agreements on issues can be discovered (if only the reader searches hard enough).

Given the opinions above, one can imagine our surprise when, upon reading the papers in this issue, we realized that they did indeed address common issues and that many important points of agreement had emerged. We will try to explicate some of these issues in the following discussion. In general, they group themselves into four broad categories: (1) consideration of the currently accepted assumptions upon which most stimulation programs are based, (2) difficulties of classifying a heterogeneous population of infants, (3) conclusions from the empirical studies which have attempted to evaluate the efficacy of infant stimulation programs, and (4) suggested future directions in our thinking about and implementation of infant stimulation programs. We have attempted, at least to

Mark S. Strauss is Associate Professor and Celia A. Brownell is Assistant Professor in the Department of Psychology at the University of Pittsburgh, Pittsburgh, Pennsylvania 15260.

*133*

some extent, to identify which papers contributed to each of the respective issues; however, since so many issues were raised in common, such credits to the authors may not be fully inclusive. That should not be taken, though, as a reflection of our opinion about the quality of any particular paper. Overall, we felt the quality was quite good, particularly in an area often marked by lack of empirical or conceptual rigor, and an area of expertise still in its own infancy.

## CURRENT ASSUMPTIONS ABOUT INFANT STIMULATION

Many of the papers including Brownell and Strauss, Casto and White, Gardner, Karmel and Down, and Ramey and Suarez discussed the fact that infant stimulation programs are typically built upon a common set of assumptions regarding the role of early experience and its effects upon later development. As Ramey and Suarez indicate, these "early experience" assumptions have long standing historical roots. Unfortunately, many of the authors also indicate that these assumptions may not have much validity. Some of these assumptions, tacitly accepted by individuals involved in infant stimulation, include:

1. there are critical periods for certain behaviors which may lead to irreversible consequences;
2. environmental factors have a greater impact on early development than do biological or hereditary factors;
3. early experiences have a direct and causal influence on later functioning, thus the earlier one intervenes, the better;
4. the effects of early stimulation are dramatic and long term;
5. relatively minor changes in an infant's environment may lead to major changes in ultimate developmental outcome;
6. as in medicine, "an ounce of prevention is worth a pound of cure."

While several of the empirical review papers (e.g., Casto and White; Bricker; Bryant and Ramey) have begun to study the validity of these claims, it is clear that much more research is needed. More important is the suggestion made by a number of the authors that there are reasons to begin to question such assumptions, and that there may be alternative views upon which infant stimulation programs can be based. As Ramey and Suarez state, "we are witnessing an attempt to retreat to an earlier but inadequate paradigm. What is needed, however, is to move forward to a more comprehensive and adequate worldview. We need a new paradigm to provide a more realistic set of expectations about human development in general and early education in particular.''

## HETEROGENEITY OF POPULATIONS

Evident from several of the papers is the fact that infant stimulation programs are directed toward a number of quite different populations. Four populations were the major focus of these papers: (1) infants who are at risk primarily because they come from disadvantaged environments and/or have inadequately prepared, teenage parents (Bryant and Ramey; Casto and White; McDonough); (2) infants who are medically at risk as a result of pre-, peri-, or post-natal complications such as prematurity (Bricker; Bryant and Ramey; Gardner, Karmel and Dowd); (3) infants who have definitive handicaps or brain-damage (Bricker); and (4) normal infants (Brownell and Strauss; Gardner et al.).

Initially these populations may appear to be relatively distinct. However, as became apparent from the articles, such distinctions are often made to aid programmatic research, and in fact may not accurately represent the real status of the populations targeted. For example, while it is possible to identify infants who may be at risk due to environmental factors, these negative environmental factors often result in the emergence of biological or physiological risk factors such as low birth weight or prematurity. Similarly, although an attempt is often made to separate infants who are biologically at risk from infants who demonstrate definitive symptoms of neurologic damage (e.g., ventricular bleeds, cerebral palsy, etc.) such distinctions can become blurred due to still limited diagnostic abilities. That is, an infant who does not demonstrate major symptoms of neurologic damage may nonetheless have more subtle damage, perhaps biochemical in nature. Finally, the distinction between "normal" and "at-risk" is often not clear. Indeed, it is perhaps best to recognize that there is probably a "continuum of biological and environmental risk factors" rather than distinct categories. Unfortunately this makes the task of conducting research and of providing intervention much more difficult since, on the one hand, our goal is to provide intervention specific to particular types of problems, yet, on the other hand, our ability to identify which types of problems are functionally or etiologically similar is still extremely limited.

## RESEARCH ON THE EFFICACY
## OF INFANT STIMULATION/INTERVENTION

Several of the articles were concerned with the empirical literature directed at determining how effective infant stimulation programs are. Casto and White conducted a "meta-analysis" of a number of published investigations in order to determine the extent to which intervention versus control subjects have differed on various developmental outcome measures. Similarly, Bryant and Ramey, Bricker, and Honig all reviewed research relevant to the efficacy of infant intervention. These papers pointed to several general conclusions:

1. Most intervention programs tend to produce only *moderate* gains in the experimental groups. These gains typically represent an improvement of about half a standard deviation.
2. There is little support for the idea that "the earlier intervention is begun, the better." Indeed, intervention begun with 2 or 3 year olds tended to be more effective than intervention that was begun in the first year of life.
3. There is little evidence of long-term effects resulting from infant stimulation/intervention.
4. The vast majority of evaluations have focused on intellectual or cognitive development and relatively few studies have measured changes in either social development or parental attitudes.
5. Our ability to determine the effectiveness of infant stimulation is extremely hindered by the lack of good predictive indices of development (which may be due to the nature of development itself, and not to the adequacy of the measures). Since most current measures derive from normal populations, this becomes more problematic when attempting to assess infants who are handicapped or medically at risk.
6. Deriving an accurate picture of the effects of infant stimulation on development is also limited by the diversity of programs, problems of population identification, and the difficulties of defining adequate control groups.

Although these summary statements suggest that infant stimulation appears to be of only limited benefit, there does appear to be hope for the future. Research on the cognitive, biological and social development of children within the first two or three years of life is still relatively new. While substantial gains in knowledge have accrued during the last ten years, the field is still in its infancy relative to most other areas of psychology. As our understanding of early development increases, it will be possible to construct intervention programs which are based more closely on known principles of development, i.e., that are appropriately timed and that are geared to specific developmental problems that are malleable or perhaps even preventable.

## FUTURE DIRECTIONS

Individuals responsible for actually developing and managing infant intervention programs may have been disappointed by the nature of the suggestions proposed in this set of papers. Concluding comments have been rather general, and little specific advice has been offered regarding program content or goals. There were no recipes for success in this special issue. However, that should be taken as an indication of just how premature it would be to attempt to provide a "cookbook" on how to set up and run an infant intervention program. More important than providing a cookbook, the papers in this volume have provided perspective on the problems of current programs, and have pointed to a number of themes that must be incorporated in the development of a framework for the future of infant intervention. These themes include the following:

1. The need for a greater emphasis on social development. Most programs have focused only on the infant's cognitive abilities. However, cognitive growth does not occur in a vacuum. To try to separate the infant's intellectual growth from his or her social environment is both artificial and counter-productive. Thus several authors make a plea for future programs to be much more comprehensive in nature. Both intervention and assessment must put more focus on social competence, parent-child relations, and the broader environmental context in which the infant is developing.
2. Not only must future programs become more comprehensive

with respect to content, they must also be more comprehensive with respect to time. Many of the authors note that it is not surprising that the effects of intervention wash out over time. Development is a continuous, ongoing process. Old models based on simple and direct causal links between early experiences and later development are just not adequate. Thus we must view infant intervention as merely a first step in a continuing program of help for both the child and his or her parents.

3. Current assessment instruments are inadequate for the purposes of infant intervention. Most infant assessment measures are product oriented. That is, they are concerned with measuring individual differences in infant outcomes with little concern given for measuring what processes are developing and how. If one accepts the view that development is a continuing and constantly changing process, then one must have a way of measuring this changing process. Fortunately, the last 20 years have seen a growing research literature on how basic sensory, perceptual, cognitive and social processes develop in the infant. These new methodologies need to be incorporated into infant intervention assessments.

4. Much more careful thought must be given to population definition and identification. It is no longer adequate to group *all* types of infants who may be at risk for later development into a single program or research project. Rather, serious thought must be given to the particular problems which may affect the pattern or process of development of different populations of at-risk infants.

5. Finally, thought should be given to the possibility that, as Gardner et al. state, "more stimulation is not necessarily better and can, in fact, be detrimental." Research with both animals and infants demonstrates that unless stimulation is "appropriate to (the infant's) developmental stage, state modulating characteristics, and capabilities" more harm than good can be accomplished.

Infant intervention/stimulation programs have been emerging at a staggering rate over the last 10 years. Tremendous investments of time and money have been made in the belief that the development of a child can be "maximized" by intervention, as early as feasible. However, as with any new area, it is vital to step back occasionally and to evaluate one's accomplishments, and only then to plan future investments firmly based upon these evaluations. The papers in this issue represent a first step at such an evaluative process. Hopefully, they will also have some impact upon the future direction of infant stimulation and intervention.

# SELECTED READINGS

## Documents and Journal Articles From The Eric Database

### ERIC DOCUMENTS

BIRTH CONDITIONS ASSOCIATED WITH MENTAL STATES AT AGE SIX, by Lawrence Hartlage and others. (1983, 22p., ED 227 968)

Reports a longitudinal study of 41 children from a high-risk neonatal nursery. Measures of neonatal condition (e.g., head size, delivery mode, etc.) were related to children's performance at age 6 on several tests of mental status. Results suggested that certain neonatal conditions may affect specific aspects of mental function more than they affect global aspects of mental status.

THE EFFECTIVENESS OF THERAPEUTIC INTERVENTION WITH INFANTS WHO HAVE CEREBRAL PALSY OR MOTOR DELAY, by Howard P. Parette, Jr., and Jack Hourcade. (1982, 21p., ED 234 524)

Eighteen studies, conducted from 1952 to 1982, are reviewed in order to evaluate early therapeutic interventions. An overview of findings suggests that, as research paradigms become more rigorous in terms of design and statistical analysis, empirical documentation of program efficacy becomes less likely.

INFANTS AT RISK: ASSESSMENT AND INTERVENTION. AN UPDATE FOR HEALTH-CARE PROFESSIONALS AND PARENTS. PEDIATRIC ROUND TABLE: 5, Edited by Catherine Caldwell Brown. (1981, 150p., ED 233 785)

Summarizes conference presentations focusing on new approaches to developmental screening of infants and strategies for early intervention with children at risk. Among the summaries are discussions of an "optimality scale" for neurological investigation and descriptions of programs for infants at risk for specific outcomes.

ISSUES IN NEONATAL CARE, Edited by Arnold Waldstein and others. (1982, 157 p., ED 224 588)

Collects articles evolved from presentations made at a workshop entitled "The Health Care/Education Relationship: Services for Infants with Special Needs and Their Families," held for members of the Handicapped Children's Early Education Program (HCEEP) network. Papers, grouped into three sections, offer remarks by leading researchers in the field, focus on the evolving role of the infant developmental specialist, and discuss innovative approaches for improving the relations between parents and professionals.

MINIMIZING HIGH-RISK PARENTING: A REVIEW OF WHAT IS KNOWN AND CONSIDERATION OF APPROPRIATE PREVENTIVE INTERVENTION, Pediatric Round Table: 7. Edited by Valerie J. Sasserath and others. (1983, 127p., ED 233 787)

Presents conference papers and discussions intended to provide a guide for intervention by health professionals and others concerned with high-risk parenting situations. Contents focus on how interventions associated with parenting can be more effectively managed to help the child and how more effective communication between parent and professional can be attained.

## JOURNAL ARTICLES

BABIES AT DOUBLE HAZARD: EARLY DEVELOPMENT OF INFANTS AT BIOLOGIC AND SOCIAL RISK, by Sibylle K. Escalona. *Pediatrics,* 1982, *70*(5), 670-676.

Reports a study of the interaction of biological and social factors on the mental and psychological development of 114 low-birth-weight premature infants from primarily poor and nonwhite urban areas. It was suggested that premature infants are more vulnerable to environmental insufficiencies than are full-term babies.

CURRENT CONCERNS OF EARLY CHILDHOOD EDU-CATORS: A CONVERSATION WITH DIANE BRICKER, by Angele M. Thomas. *Education and Training of the Mentally Retarded,* 1982, *17*(2), 114-119.

Interview questions focus on such questions as the effect of federal cutbacks for early childhood education, status of main-streaming for preschoolers, effective intervention models, successful parent involvement, curriculum development and evaluation, and learning in the at-risk infant.

THE DEVELOPMENTALIST AND THE STUDY OF BIOLOGI-CAL RISK: A VIEW OF THE PAST WITH AN EYE TOWARD THE FUTURE, by Claire B. Kopp and Joanne B. Krakow. *Child Development,* 1983, *54*(5), 1086-1108.

Examines the history of the developmental study of infants and children at biological risk, and appraises the current state of the science. Four research phases during the period from 1920 to the present are identified; each reflects aspects of the social, political, health, and psychological zeitgeist.

EVIDENCE FOR PREVENTION OF DEVELOPMENTAL RE-
TARDATION DURING INFANCY, by Craig T. Ramey and Don-
na M. Bryant. *Journal of the Division for Early Education,* 1982, *5,*
73-38.

Reviews children's intellectual response to four major programs
concerned with the prevention of developmental retardation. (The
programs surveyed used experimentally adequate research designs.)

HIGH-RISK INFANTS OF TEENAGE MOTHERS: LATER
CANDIDATES FOR SPECIAL EDUCATION PLACEMENTS?,
by Elizabeth Landerholm. *Journal of the Division for Early Childhood,* 1982, *6,* 3-13.

Provides an overview of research on teenage pregnancy, the
special educational needs of the infants of these teenage mothers,
and current intervention programs for teenage mothers and their infants. The research demonstrates that intervention programs can affect infant mortality, morbidity, and prematurity as well as social
and cognitive development.

ERIC, the Educational Resources Information Center, is funded
by the National Institute of Education, U.S. Department of Education. Within the ERIC system are 16 separate clearinghouses, each
responsible for collecting and disseminating information on a
specific subject area in education. The ERIC Clearinghouse on
Elementary and Early Childhood Education (ERIC/EECE) deals
with information relating to the education and development of children from birth through age 12.

ERIC DOCUMENTS (those with ED numbers) are cited and
abstracted in the monthly index *Resources in Education (RIE).* The
majority of these documents may be read on microfiche at the many
libraries and information service agencies housing ERIC microfiche
collections. In addition, most are available on microfiche or in paper
copy from the ERIC Document Reproduction Service, P.O. Box
190, Arlington, VA 22210. Since prices are subject to change,
please contact ERIC/EECE or consult the most recent issue of *RIE*
for ordering information.

JOURNAL ARTICLES are cited and annotated in the monthly publication *Current Index to Journals in Education (CIJE)*. These articles may be read in periodicals obtained in libraries or through subscription. Selected article reprints are available from University Microfilms International, Article Reprint Department, 300 N. Zeeb Road, Ann Arbor, MI 48106. Please contact ERIC/EECE or see the most recent issue of *CIJE* for UMI ordering details.

Further information about the ERIC network and services of the ERIC Clearinghouse on Elementary and Early Childhood Education are available from ERIC/EECE Information Services, College of Education, University of Illinois, 805 W. Pennsylvania Ave., Urbana, IL 61801 (Telephone: 217-333-1386).